Cosmetic Surgery

Edited by Yueh-Bih Tang

Published in London, United Kingdom

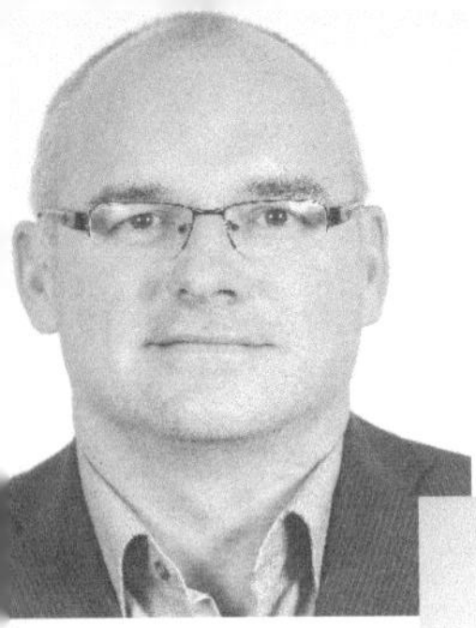
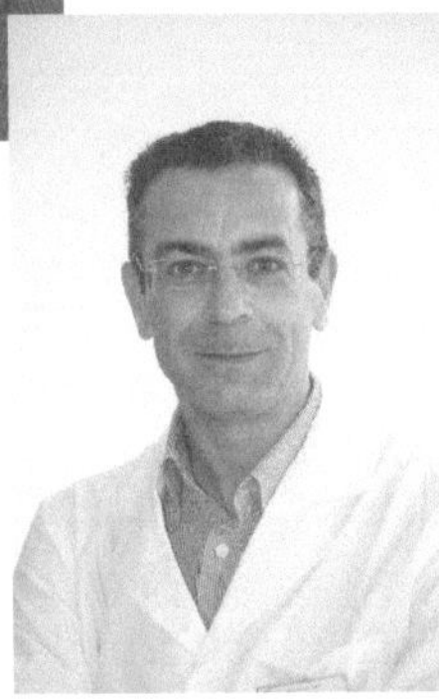
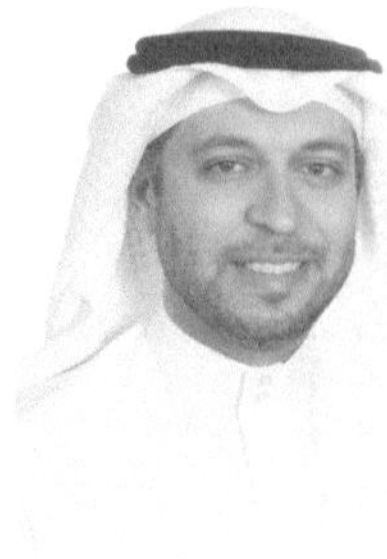
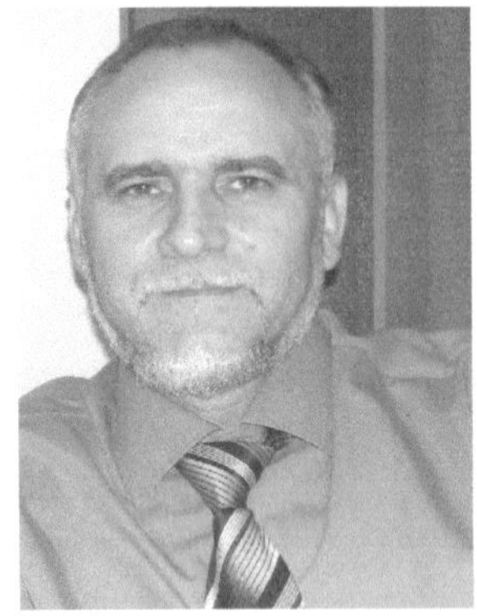
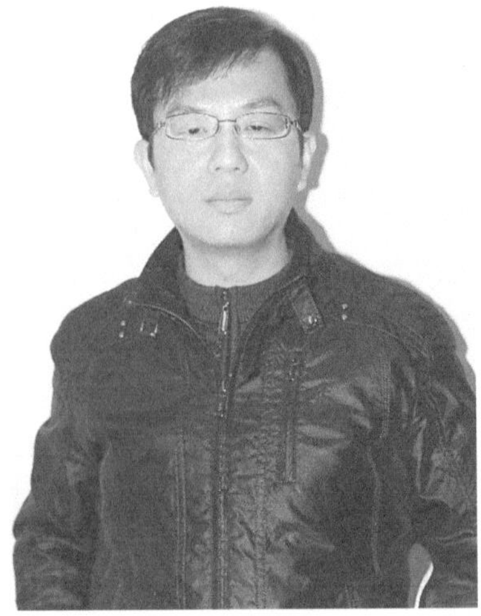
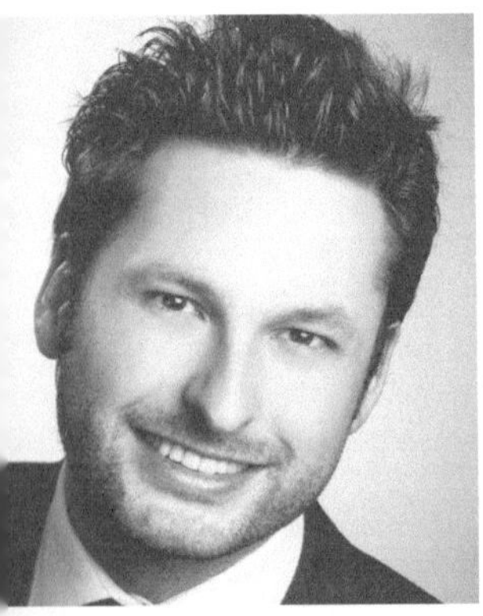
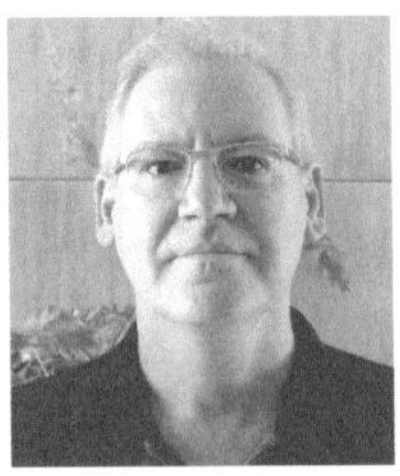

IntechOpen

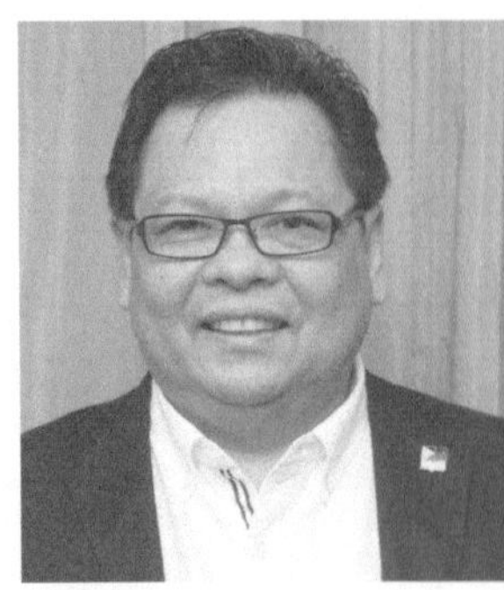
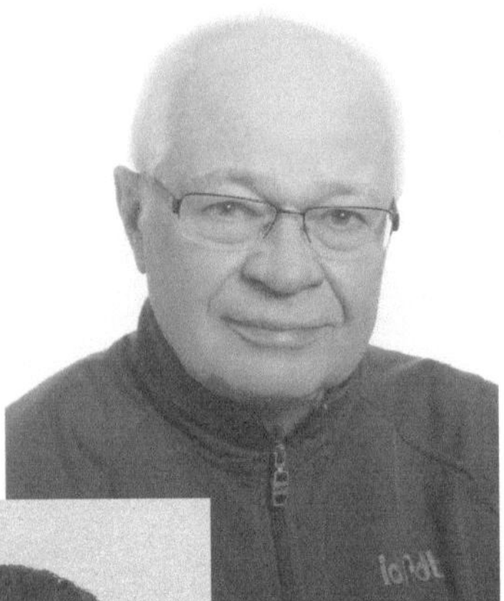
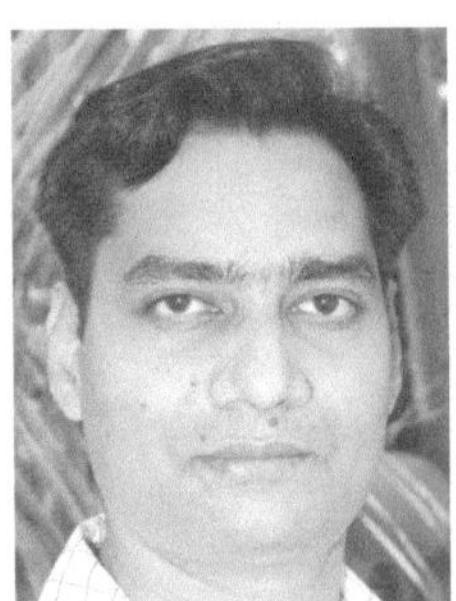
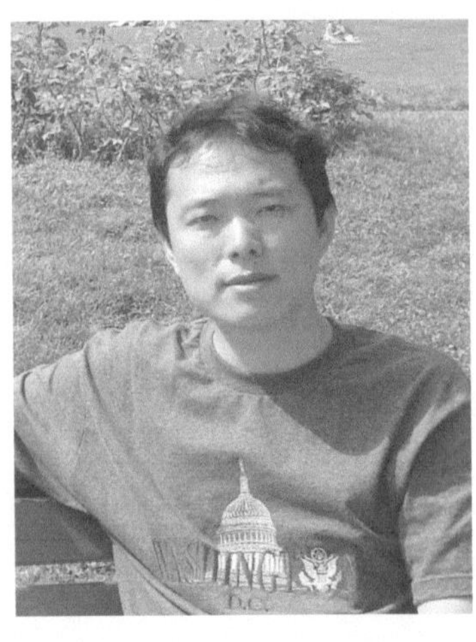
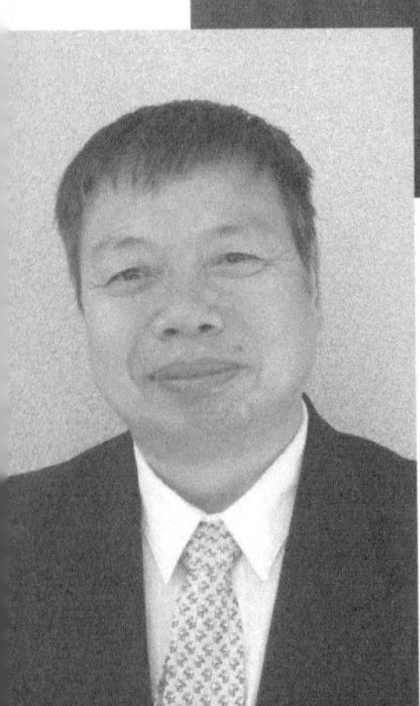
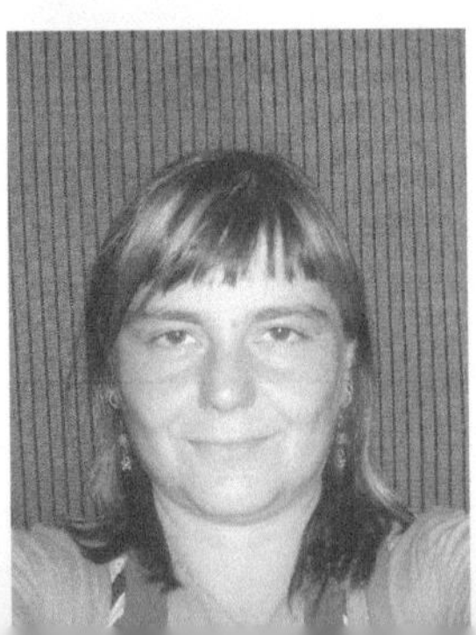

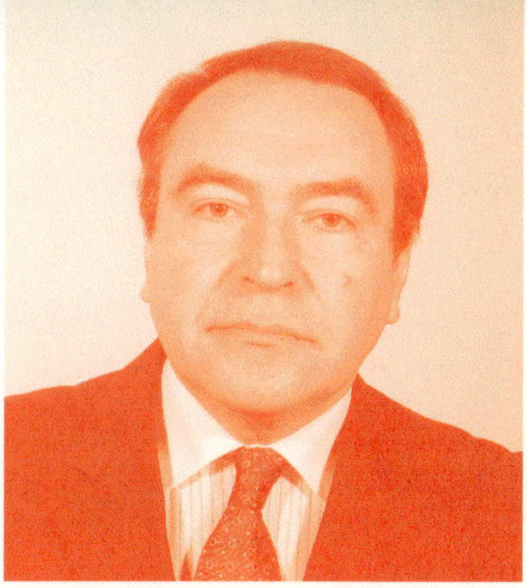
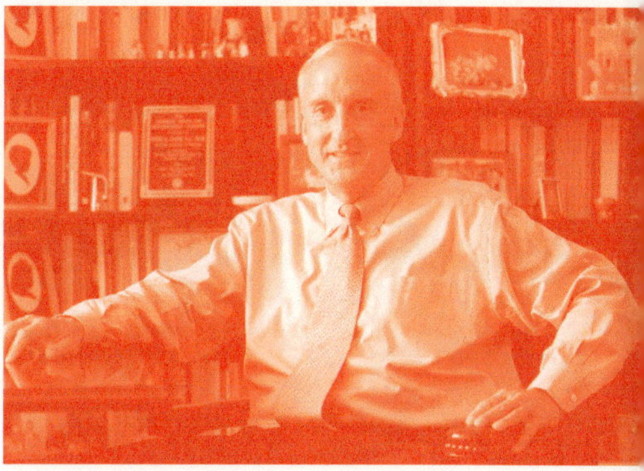
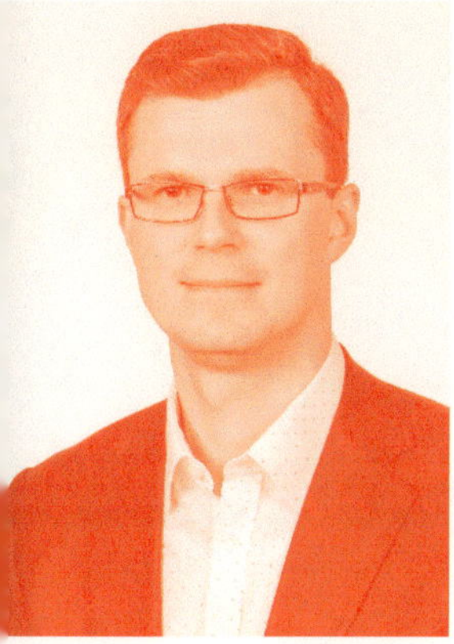
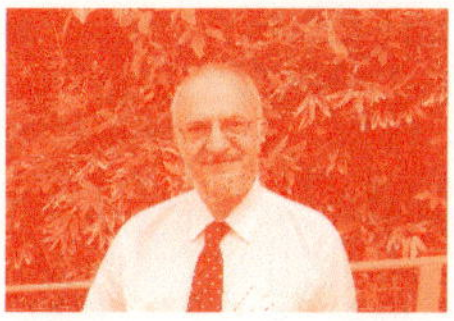
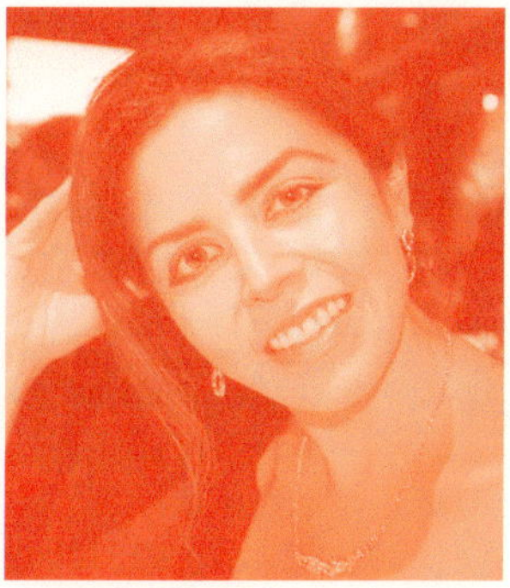

Supporting open minds since 2005

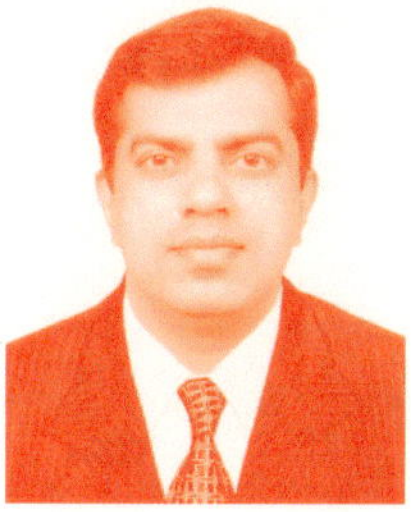
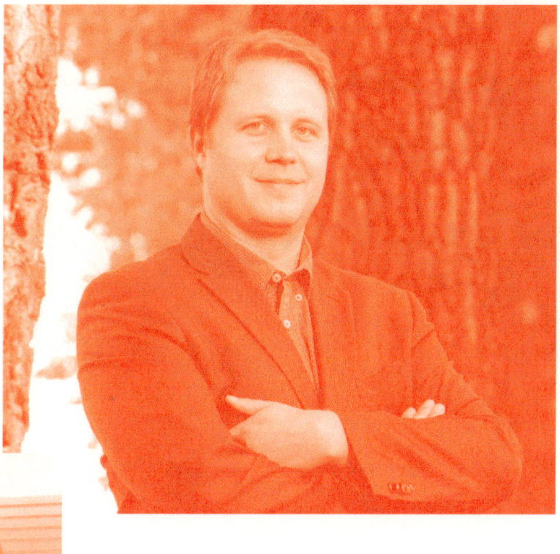
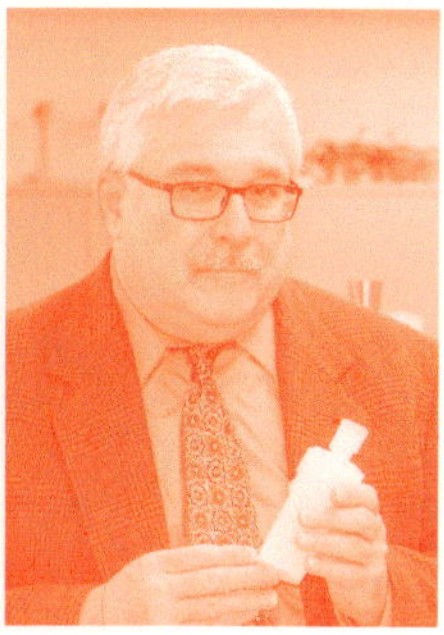
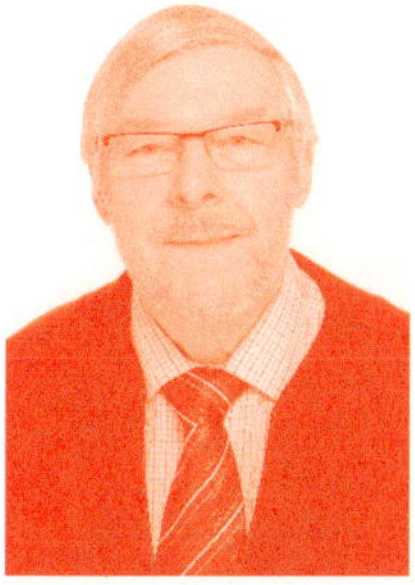
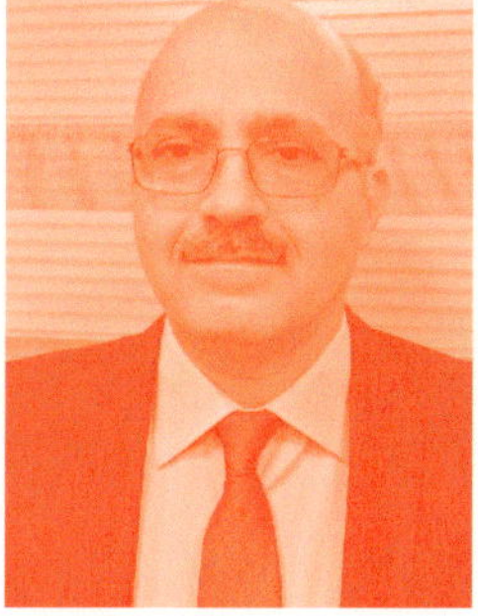
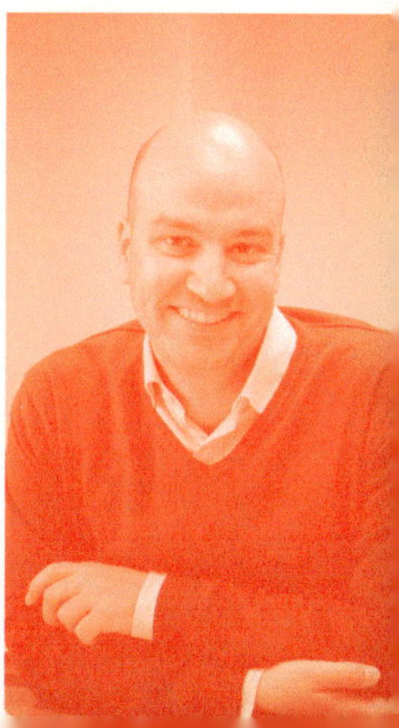
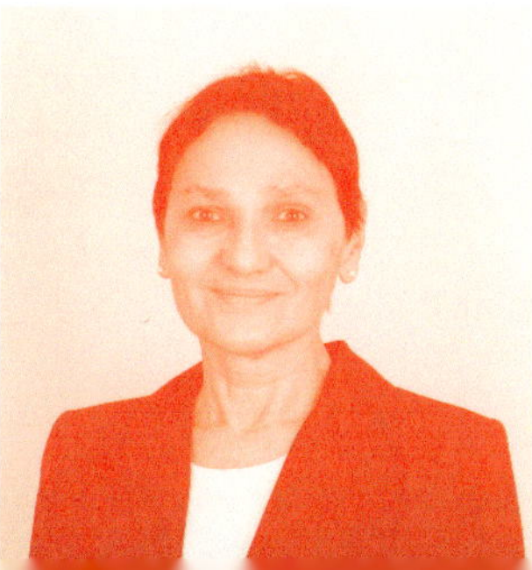

Cosmetic Surgery
http://dx.doi.org/10.5772/intechopen.83118
Edited by Yueh-Bih Tang

Contributors
Ago Harlim, Chuan-Hsiang Kao, Sarina Rajbhandari, Amin Amer, Diane Irvine Duncan, Mohamed Amer, Hagar Nofal

First published in London, United Kingdom, 2021 by IntechOpen
IntechOpen is the global imprint of INTECHOPEN LIMITED, registered in England and Wales, registration number: 11086078, 5 Princes Gate Court, London, SW7 2QJ, United Kingdom
Printed in Croatia

British Library Cataloguing-in-Publication Data
A catalogue record for this book is available from the British Library

Additional hard and PDF copies can be obtained from orders@intechopen.com

Cosmetic Surgery
Edited by Yueh-Bih Tang
p. cm.
Print ISBN 978-1-83880-367-4
Online ISBN 978-1-83880-368-1
eBook (PDF) ISBN 978-1-83881-218-8

Meet the editor

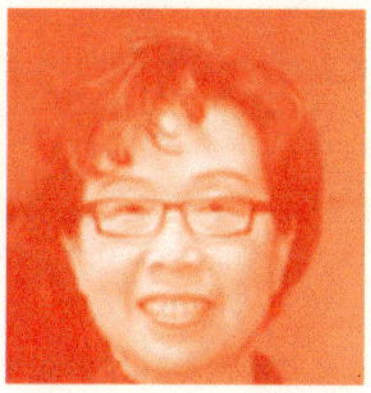

Yueh-Bih Tang is a Professor in plastic surgery at the National Taiwan University Hospital, Taipei, Taiwan. She is also the Director of the Center for Human Appearance, Far-Eastern Memorial Hospital, Banqiao, New Taipei City, Taiwan. She is a past President of the Taiwan Society of Plastic Surgery, as well as a past President of the Taiwan Society of Aesthetic Plastic.

Contents

Preface

This edited volume is a collection of reviewed and relevant research chapters concerning the developments within the Cosmetic Surgery field of study. The book includes scholarly contributions by various authors and it has been edited by a group of experts pertinent to medicine. Each contribution comes as a separate chapter complete in itself but directly related to the book's topics and objectives.

The book contains the following chapters: "Management of Nasal Silicone Granuloma", "Costal Cartilage Graft in Asian Rhinoplasty: Surgical Techniques", "Botulinum Toxin for the Face", "Combining Helium Plasma-Driven Radiofrequency with Nanofat for Contouring", and "Combining PDO Threads with Exosomes for Microlifting".

The target audience comprises scholars and specialists in the field.

IntechOpen

Chapter 1

Management of Nasal Silicone Granuloma

Ago Harlim

Abstract

The use of silicone as filler material has been banned by the FDA. Nevertheless, there are still some risks of using topical silicone, particularly cosmetic products that contain silicone. Bioavailability of silicone in skin tissues and long-term complications of silicone use in cosmetic products must be evaluated for safety reasons. Silicone can penetrate to the skin by injection. Because of economic issues and the rarity of medical grade silicone, various developing countries use industrial silicone, which results in even more complications. Patients with liquid silicone injected to their nose will usually visit a doctor after experiencing complication issues such as granuloma, edema, and redness with telangiectasia. Usually the patients want to remove the silicone and treat the complication. Unfortunately, silicone is difficult to be removed completely. Some complications are difficult to treat. To handle this complication issue, the doctor has to create a specific design of nose implant, perform curettage, or remove silicone and granuloma, and then a laser treatment and steroid injection will be performed.

Keywords: silicone, skin, topical, nasal implant, laser

1. Introduction

Silicone injection has been used since 40 years ago, and at that time, many problems occurred such as migration, inflammation, and granuloma. In 1992, the FDA prohibited silicone injection for cosmetic use [1]. In addition to injection, silicone may be introduced into our body or skin through food intake and cosmetic. Silicone has been widely used in daily cosmetics. Nowadays, due to technology advances, topical drugs can pass through skin barrier and can be penetrated into the skin, which has become a great concern as it may induce granuloma formation. There are relatively very few studies that have been done on silicone concentration in the normal skin.

A study conducted by Harlim in 2018 found that a normal skin contained silicon. The study was performed by taking skin samples from normal subjects and those with face-lift procedure and subsequently compared those samples using the same criteria with the control group, which included skin samples of subjects that had received silicone injection, and the study found granuloma formation. The study found an average amount of silicon level of 44.07 ± 75.86 μg/g in patients with normal skin, while in patients with granuloma, they found 38 times greater silicon level (1709.21 ± 1851.72 μg/g) [2].

IntechOpen

2. Silicone

Injectable-grade silicone for medical use has been manufactured widely since the element has been known for its stable and inert characteristics [3, 4]. It includes the use of silicone oil, which has been utilized in the treatment of complicated retinal detachment and heavy silicone oil tamponade. The treatment seems to offer promising results, particularly on improving visual acuity as well as great results on some anatomical parameters; however, there are some concerns as it may cause several complications such as cataract, increased ocular pressure, heavy silicone oil emulsification, and mild inflammatory reaction [5–7].

Injectable-grade silicone has also been widely used in the form of silicone oil injection. Some studies have suggested that it may have an essential role in reducing the risk of developing diabetic foot ulcer due to its pressure-reducing properties; therefore, it can maintain plantar tissue thickness and alleviate symptoms of diabetic foot ulcer, which may be associated with foot biomechanics [8, 9].

Although it brings advantages, silicone injection may still develop some complications, either local or systemic complications. Local complications may include formation of palpable nodule surrounding injection site, arthralgia, fatigue, electrical neuropathy, and electrical sensation [10], while systemic complications may also occur in the form of lymphadenopathy, renal disease, and hepatic disease. It indicates that the injected silicone can migrate from injection site to other organs causing local and systemic complications. An animal experimental study in mouse model may explain the pathogenesis of such complications. The study has demonstrated that macrophage of skin tissue may engulf the injected silicone and the silicone may be distributed through lymphatic circulation, ultimately causing accumulation in lymph nodes, adrenal glands, and the kidney, liver, and spleen as well as granuloma formation in the skin [11]. Complications due to silicone injection, particularly the granuloma formation may be dose-dependent. A study by Harlim has demonstrated that granuloma formation could be developed when there is a large amount of silicone exposure as the study only found a low level of silicone without any granuloma formation in the normal skin (**Figure 1**) [2].

Cultural changes have been encouraging people to pursue their passion on beauty and youth; therefore, cosmeticology has been rapidly growing. With technological advances, more mixed drug ingredients have been added to cosmetic products in order to beautify their customers. Thus, it may indirectly increase the use of topical

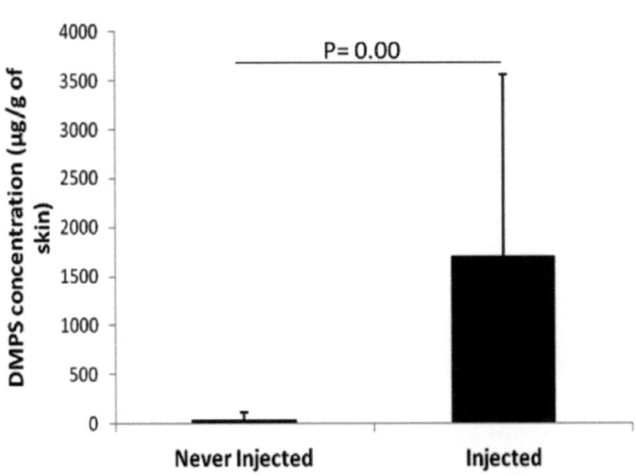

Figure 1.
The level of silicon (Si) in normal subjects who had never received silicone injection (never injected) and in subjects with granuloma who had received silicone injection. (cited from A Harlim, et all) [2].

cosmetics that usually contain silicone; therefore, it will lead to increase silicone uptake to the skin. It has raised a concern that the prolonged and continuous use of cosmetics will cause granuloma formation and other chronic inflammatory effects.

3. Dietary intake and silicon

Aside from medical use, silicon has also been used in food industry, cosmetics, and pharmaceutical industries. Our data shows that the silicon levels in gastrointestinal medications (e.g., antacids), mineral water, and soda drinks are 44.1, 25.6, and 2.91 μg/g, respectively. It can be said that there are many routes for administering silicon into our body. The average daily intake of silicon for European and North American populations is 20–50 mg/day. In China and India, the daily intake of silicon is larger that may reach as many as 140–200 mg/day, in which wheats, fruits, and vegetables are the greatest producers [12].

A research institution of healthy aging and nutrition in the United Kingdom has recently reported a strong correlation between silicon in dietary intake and the health of bone and connective tissue. Therefore, it can be assumed that the correlation is associated with collagen synthesis and/or stabilization of mineral matrix, i.e., silicone intake may affect bone density [13].

Another study, which is an animal experimental study, has demonstrated that there is no evidence of silicon accumulation in silicon consumption. Silicon can be eliminated through digestion process and can be found in feces (93–97%), urine (0.001–0.22%), and expired air (0.01–0.02%) [3]. It indicates that silicon is a stable element and at certain degree it can be resistant to digestive enzymes including gastric acid; therefore, it seems that silicon is not accumulated in the gastroinstestinal system.

4. Silicone in cosmetics

Beauty products for face, hair, and cosmetics may have high silicone content, in which it will be accumulated in the skin tissue. When a topical beauty product containing silicone is applied to the skin, the elastomeric particles of silicone will absorb various liquids including emollient and oil; therefore, silicone is used in skin care product as vehicle (carrier) of active ingredient for the skin or as oil control product of the skin [4, 5].

Types of silicone that are commonly used in cosmetic products:

- Dimethicone—clear, inert, liquid solubility depends on the length of polymer backbone ranging in thickness from watery consistency to thick.
- Dimethicone copolyol—silicone that contains an —OH group; therefore, it is more water-soluble resulting in easier incorporation into water-based formulations and also reduces the "slip effect" of the silicone.
- Cyclomethicone—the shortest cyclic molecule, which has many similarities with dimethicone except it can evaporate, while dimethicone cannot.
- Cyclo-dimethicone—a combination of dimethicone and cyclomethicones.

The great use of silicones in cosmetic product may increase the risk of accumulation of the substance in our body, particularly in the facial skin. No clear evidence has been found on the bioavailability and concentration of accumulated silicone in topical uses.

5. Granuloma: definition

Granuloma is a foreign body reaction against foreign substances that enter the skin. Granuloma occurs due to continuous or chronic inflammation against foreign substances. Silicone is a foreign substance in the body, which will be encapsulated by the body. Datia cells (giant cells) will encapsulate silicone material, and therefore inflammatory mediators cannot perform phagocytosis, which results in continuous inflammation and causes side effect. The encapsulated material has poor vascularization; therefore, it may potentially induce infections [6].

6. Classification and etiology

There are many kinds of granuloma classification; however, the common classifications are those which have been adjusted to the etiologies [7, 8]. Granuloma formation may occur due to various factors such as biologic, chemical, and physical irritative agents [7]. Classification based on clinical, etiological, and histopathological features

Infections	**Immunological aberration**
Fungi	Sarcoidosis
Histoplasma	Crohn's disease
Coccidioides	Primary biliary cirrhosis
Blastomyces	Giant cell arteritis
Sporothrix	Peyronie's disease
Aspergillus	Hypogammaglobulinemia
Cryptococcus	Langerhans' granulomatosis
	Hepatic granulomatous disease
	Immune complex disease
Protozoa	
Interferon-δ-receptor deficiency	
Toxoplasma	
Leishmania	
	Vasculitic granulomatosis
Metazoa	Wegener's
Toxocara	Necrotizing sarcoidal
Schistosoma	Churg-Strauss
	Lymphomatoid
Spirochaetes	Polyarteritis nodosa
T. Pallidum	Bronchocentric
T. carateum	Systemic lupus
T. pertune	
Mycobacteria	**Leukocyte oxidase defect**
M. tuberculosis	Chronic granulomatous
M. leprae	disease of childhood

Infections	**Immunological aberration**
M. kansasii	
M. marinum	**Hypersensitivity pneumonitis**
M. avian	Farmers' lung
BCG vaccine	Bird fanciers'
	Mushroom workers'
Bacteria	Suberosis (cork dust)
Brucella	Bagassosis
Yersinia	Maple bark strippers'
	Paprika splitters'
Other infections	Coffee bean
Cat-scratch	Spatlese lung
Lymphogranuloma	
	Other
Neoplasia	Fibrosing alveolitis
Carcinoma	Whipple's disease
Reticulosis	Pyrexia of unknown origin
Pinealoma	Radiotherapy
Dysgerminoma	Cancer chemotherapy
Seminoma	Panniculitis
Reticulum cell sarcoma	Chalazion
Malignant nasal granuloma	Sebacous cyst
	Dermoid
Chemicals	Sea urchin spine injury
Beryllium	Tattoo
Zirconium	Malakoplakia
Silica	Blau's syndrome
Starch	

Table 1.
Classification of granulomatous disorders (cited from James DG, Wiliams WL) [8].

can be categorized further into infection, vasculitis, immunological aberration, leukocyte oxidation deficiency, hypersensitivity, chemicals, or neoplasma [14, 15]. **Table 1** presents classification of granuloma based on etiology [8].

7. Silicone granuloma

Silicone granuloma is a foreign body granuloma, which is characterized by the presence of multinuclear Datia cells and macrophages surrounded by lymphocytes and infiltrates of neutrophils. The granulomatous histological lesion caused by silicone varies depending on the type of silicone.

Tissue reactions to silicone gel or liquids are characterized by the formation of silicone granuloma with cystic space containing foreign body [9]. The irregular surface of silicone cannot be phagocytosed completely by macrophage. Datia cells are formed due to "frustrated" macrophages. Microspheres in the size of less than 15

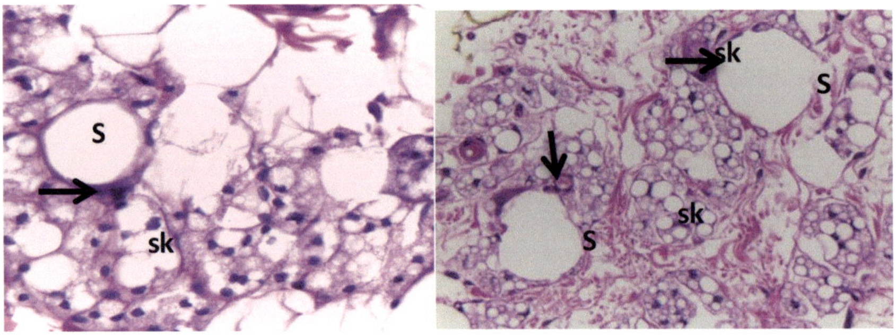

Figure 2.
Results of histopathological examination (HE 400× magnification) in one of study subject. There is a Datia cell (arrow), which is phagocytosing silicone (S) and is trying to destroy it into smaller pieces (sk) [1].

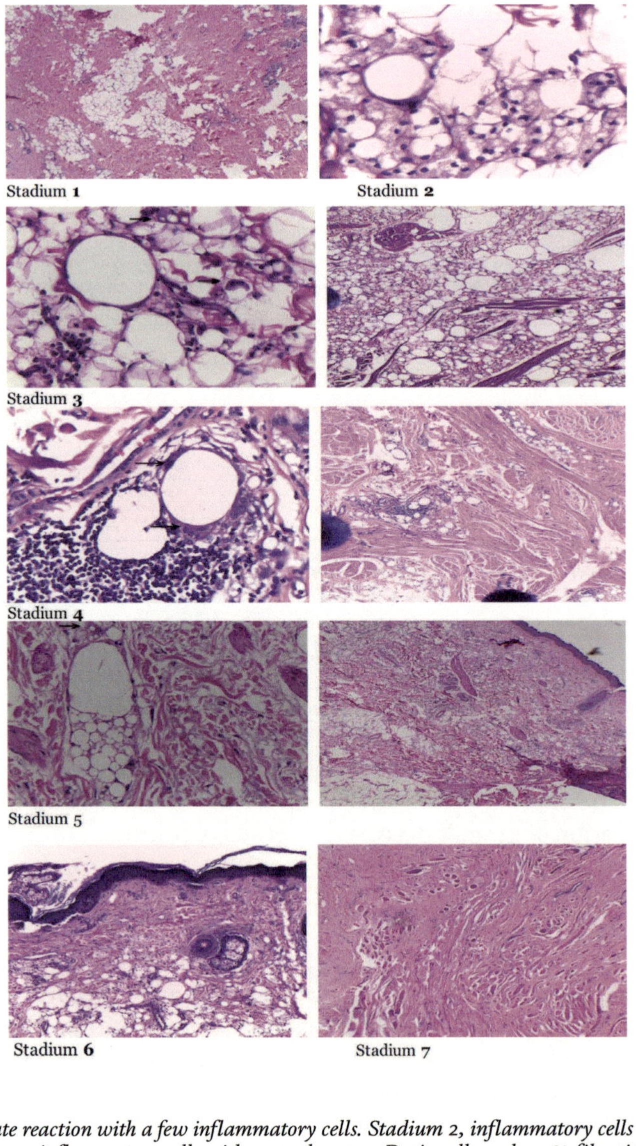

Figure 3.
Stadium 1, moderate reaction with a few inflammatory cells. Stadium 2, inflammatory cells with one or two Datia cells. Stadium 3, inflammatory cells with more than two Datia cells and <50% fibrotic area. Stadium 4, inflammatory cells with more than two Datia cells and >50% fibrotic area. Stadium 5, inflammatory cells with one Datia cell and >50% fibrotic area. Stadium 6, <50% fibrotic area with no Datia cell. Stadium 7, >50% fibrotic area with no Datia cell. (cited from A Harlim, et all) [11].

microns will be phagocytosed and transferred to the lymph node, while those with big size and nonabsorbable polymer will be encapsulated by fibrotic tissue [10].

Datia cell is essential in tissue response to silicone as seen in **Figure 2**, in which the Datia cell is phagocytosing the silicone. It appears that although the Datia cell cannot eliminate the silicone, it would produce fragmented silicone into smaller pieces. Within a month, the silicone will be in the size of 20–100 microns [11]. However, it still cannot be completely phagocytosed, and ultimately it will be encapsulated by fibrotic tissue.

In general, silicone granuloma can be categorized into three phases according to the natural history of our immune response, which are mild inflammatory phase, i.e., stage 1; inflammation with datia cells, i.e., stages 2, 3, 4, and 5; and tolerance phase with fibrosis, i.e., stages 6 and 7 (**Figure 3**).

According to Harlim in 2018, histopathological features of silicone granuloma can be categorized into seven stages, which are: [11]

Stadium 1, moderate reaction with a few inflammatory cells
Stadium 2, inflammatory cells with one or two Datia cells
Stadium 3, inflammatory cells with more than two Datia cells and <50% fibrotic area
Stadium 4, inflammatory cells with more than two Datia cells and >50% fibrotic area
Stadium 5, inflammatory cells with one Datia cell and >50% fibrotic area
Stadium 6, <50% fibrotic area with no Datia cell
Stadium 7, >50% fibrotic area with no Datia cell

8. Diagnosis

Granuloma is a form of localized nodular inflammation, which is found in tissues [7]. On examination, there is a tumor-like mass or node of granulation tissue with active fibroblast growth and capillaries that contain epithelial-like macrophages surrounded by mononuclear cells, lymphocytes, and sometime multinucleated Datia cells present at the central core of granuloma [16].

On clinical point of view, silicone granuloma is characterized by the presence of complications of silicone. There are usually granuloma nodes, migrating silicone, wider nose, and signs of inflammation such as redness and swelling depending on the stage (**Figure 4**).

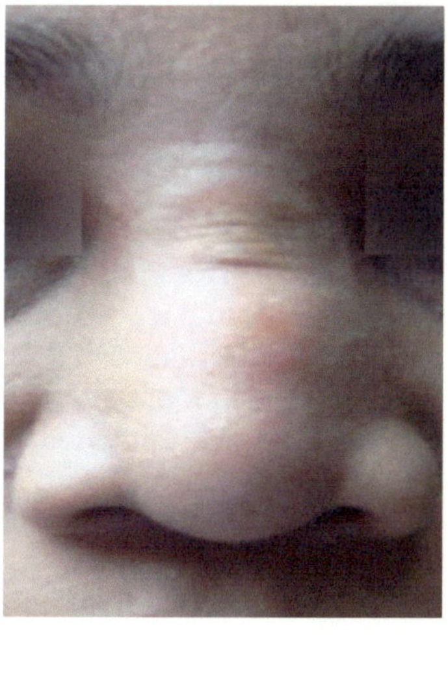

Figure 4.
Granuloma due to nasal silicone injection. The photograph shows granuloma node, migrating silicone, wider nose, and signs of inflammation such as edema and redness.

9. Management

The management of silicone-induced granuloma is often difficult due to migrating silicone and some of the silicone penetrating into the skin reaching the epidermis. In general, the management of granuloma can be categorized into two, i.e., surgical and pharmacological treatments. The management of nasal silicone granuloma is adjusted for the occurring complications. We must remove granuloma, which is under the skin; afterward, we perform excision of the excessive skin or implant insertion, creating a firmer and cosmetically more attractive skin. Remaining fibrosis or granuloma can be treated using steroid injection, and laser therapy is performed for redness.

10. Recommendation for surgical care

Granuloma formation occurs due to the presence of foreign body. Skin granuloma will cause a cosmetic problem; therefore, it should be removed.

11. Preoperative preparation

The preoperative preparation is similar to all kinds of skin surgery. A consultation prior to surgical procedure is necessary so that the doctor can perform both physical and psychological evaluation for the candidate. The patient should be informed about surgical procedure and the result may not be perfect as clean silicone injection can never be performed and there is a possibility of swelling. Patients with extreme high expectation will file their complaints in the future.

During the consultation, we must find out about coagulation disorder, either primary or secondary, either due to medication of pharmacological treatment or supplementation. The patients are advised to avoid food or medication that may prolong the bleeding time within 1 or 2 weeks prior to the procedure such as anticoagulants, aspirin, ginseng, garlic, cod liver oil, anticholesterol agent, vitamin E, warfarin, and *Ginkgo biloba*.

Curettage procedure of nasal silicone granuloma is similar to skin graft procedure, in which the covering skin must be viable. On curettage, the skin will be thinner, and it can be necrotic if there is poor vascularization. Other issues that should come into our consideration are alcohol intake, smoking habit, metabolic disorder, and poor nutrition. Blood pressure and diabetes mellitus must be well-controlled [17–19].

12. Informed consent

When a skin surgeon decides to perform a surgical procedure, both doctor and patient must consequently understand the impact, risk, and advantages of the procedure. First, the doctor needs to explain the diagnosis and the procedure that will be performed. Treatment of nasal silicone injection is a combination of medical therapy and cosmetic procedure because when it is left untreated, there will be changes such as migration, granuloma, and continuous inflammation. The risks and the advantages of the procedure should be emphasized. Moreover, the procedure during the surgery and the expected result after surgery need to be explained. Possible risks that may develop such as infection and its prevention including the use of antibiotics must also be explained. Patients must know other probable risks such as bleeding, crooked nose, wound scar that probably occurs, asymmetrical nostrils, an implant impression on the skin, granuloma or fibrosis that cannot be cleaned up, persistent redness of skin color, and other modalities of treatment that need to be carried out after the surgical procedure. It should also be explained that the results probably may be imperfect, particularly for patients with unrealistic wish. Results of discussion and patient's consent are written on an informed consent form, which is subsequently signed by the doctor and patient.

13. Technique and procedure

Every granuloma in the skin that causes cosmetic problem must be removed. Granuloma at inflammatory phase must also be removed to prevent the extension of inflammation. Local or general anesthesia could be used for procedures of skin excision, granuloma curettage, or installation of nasal implant. Instruments that must be prepared included minor surgery set, which can be equipped with curettage kit for cases that need curettage.

14. Preoperative planning

The management of silicone-induced granuloma depends on the affected area; however, basically a doctor will first make a design planning. Next, the doctor will perform procedures according to the design or images and following the plan that has been discussed with the patient.

Depending on the occurring complication, we evaluate whether we need to remove the excessive skin from the nasal columella or should only perform curettage and subsequently install a nasal implant.

Mark the area that will be excised and the protruding granuloma on the dorsal of the nose; therefore, during the surgery we emphasize on the location where the curettage will take place. If we plan to place a solid nasal implant, then we need to make a midline to ensure the implant stays straight when the swelling occurs due to anesthetic drugs.

Depending on the problem, when the nasal dorsum has become wider along with inflammation and the damaged skin, an elliptical vertical excision can be performed on it (**Figure 5**).

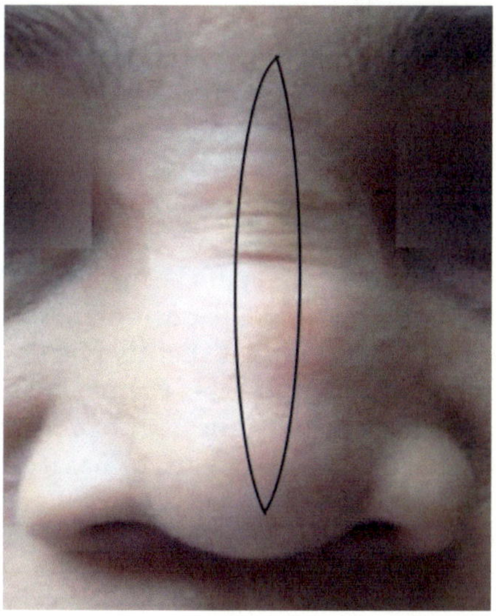

Figure 5.
Elliptical excision of granuloma on the nasal skin.

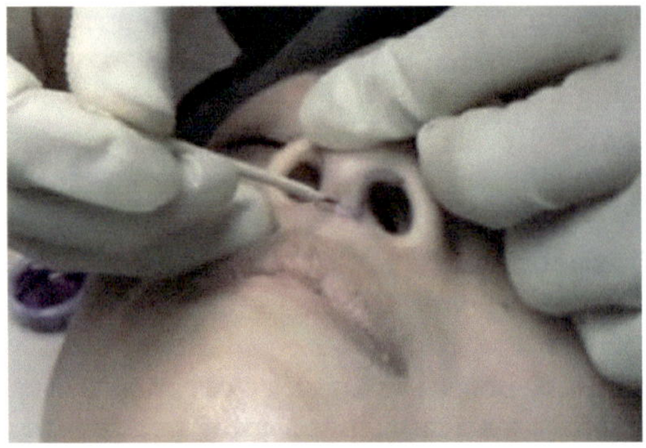

Figure 6.
Design of excision procedure to remove the excessive skin at columella area.

During silicone injection, it is common to have a wider and descending skin at the area of nasal columella due to migration of silicone injection, which always run downward from the nose; therefore, a skin excision can be performed at lateral and dorsal areas of the nasal columella (**Figure 6**).

15. Technique

After we have planned the management to overcome nasal problems, we subsequently transfer the plan into preoperative design images and subsequently perform an incision or excision following the plan.

16. Design of nasal implant

In some cases that require implants, the nasal implant is first carved before an excision is performed. Solid implant that has been commonly used is the L-shaped solid implant; however, other kinds of solid implant can also be used.

In making an implant, there are some guidelines on facial esthetics and architectural balance that should be considered.

The face can be divided into three zones with identical width. The first includes a horizontal line from the hairline to the eyebrow; the second horizontal line is from the eyebrow to the nasal base and menton; and the third horizontal line is the line from the nasal base to the end border of the chin.

The association between the lips and chin should be evaluated. The chin projection is determined by a vertical line drawn from a point of one and a half ideal length of the nose to the part of vermillion of the upper lip. The lower lip cannot be more than 2 mm posterior to this line. The position of chin varies extremely depending on sex. In women, the position is slightly posterior to the lower lips, while in men the position of the chin is in-line (**Figure 7**) [20, 21].

The implant is carved or made prior to anesthetic procedure following the guidelines of architectural balance and problems of nasal silicone granuloma as well as the patient's preferences. For nasal silicone granuloma cases, L-shaped nasal solid implant is used, and part of the nasal bridge is shaved so that it becomes slender since patients with granuloma due to silicone injection usually have wider nose and they want the nose become slender (**Figure 3**).

The height or the length of the implant is the midline border between the eye and eyebrow up to the nose. The crus of the implant must be measured following

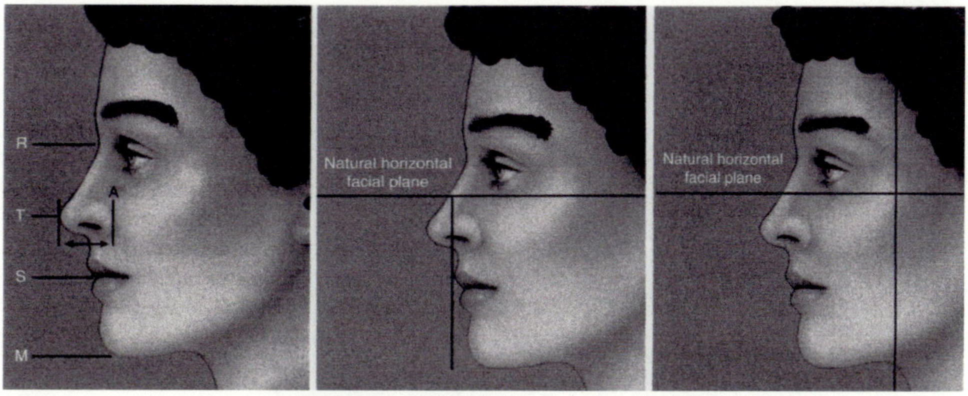

Figure 7.
Guidelines on measuring facial beauty and architectural balance.

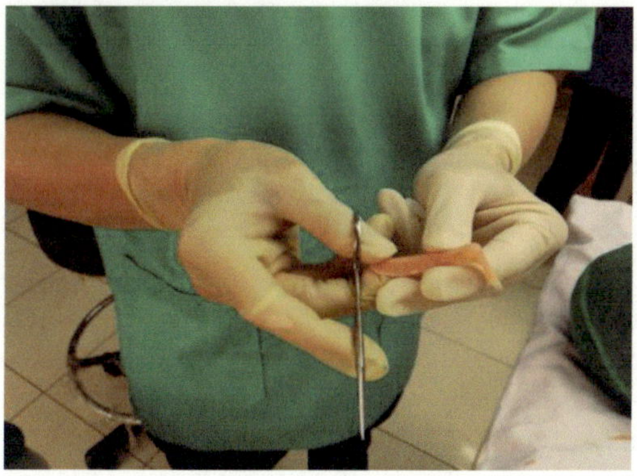

Figure 8.
L-shaped solid silicone implant. The edge is shaved so it becomes slender.

the base of columella to the nose. Usually, the crus is made straight so that it can elevate the descending skin caused by silicone injection (**Figures 8** and **9**).

Incision is always made on a hidden area and follows the contour of Langer's line. The excision is made following preoperative design image, which is an elliptical excision on the nasal dorsum (**Figure 5**); the procedure is generally performed when the condition is very severe with inflammation and the skin is wrinkled and extremely wider. The risks of the procedure are the formation of thin vertical scar line on the nasal dorsum and dog-ear phenomenon at the end of excision. An accurate calculation before surgery is essential. It is suggested that the skin removal should not be too wide to prevent dog-ear phenomenon or we can place a nasal implant so that it seems firm and creates a better look. Excision can also be made on the area adjacent to excision cut in order to reduce granuloma around the lateral nose. The skin superior to the granuloma must be thick enough to maintain vascularization and a viable skin. Many patients do not want any lengthy scar along their nose; therefore, the management of nasal silicone granuloma only includes curettage, placement of implant, and excision of the excessive skin at columella area.

After the patient received anesthetics using lidocaine or xylocaine without adrenalin, we perform a skin excision at the columella area and remove the excessive skin on the lateral and dorsal columella; afterwards, we perfom undermining procedure inferior to the granuloma using a curved clamp starting from the nasal dorsum area to the nasal bridge near the glabella and lateral of nose depending on the occurring problem. Next, curettage is performed to remove the granuloma. The skin superior

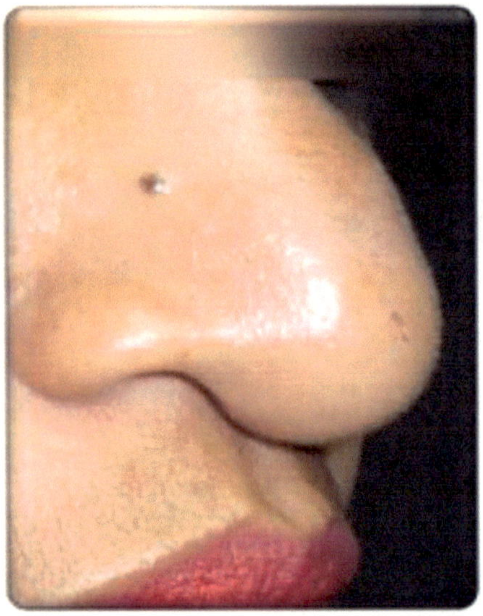

Figure 9.
Patients with silicone injection usually have wider columella area since liquid silicone will migrate downward due to gravity. Therefore, we have to remove the excessive skin of the lateral and the dorsal columella and place the implant to create a straight nose.

to it must be thick enough and well-vascularized. In cases with remaining granuloma with thick fibrosis and those with difficulty in curettage, other modalities should be performed after surgical recovery period such as steroid injection.

To create a good-shaped nose, we remove the excessive skin at the columella area, and at the nasal bridge, we can place an implant so that the skin is firmer and the shape is cosmetically better. Nasal silicone implant is placed under the nasal skin at the curettage area, which has been previously occupied by silicone granuloma.

We can perform curettage to remove silicone and granuloma. In order to create a better superior nasal tip so that the nose seems straighter, we have two choices. The first choice is that we can place the implant under the skin, and at the area, the curettage is performed; or we can put sutures at the lateral area of superior tip of the nose from lateral columella with opposite direction as presented in the following video.

17. Postoperative management

1. Use nasal splint or gauze for a week to prevent splint displacement.
2. Prescribing antibiotics for 5–7 days.
3. Prescribing analgetics every 4–6 hours as necessary.
4. Prescribing anti-inflammatory drugs for 5–7 days.
5. Normal saline solution for the nose to overcome postsurgical nasal congestion.
6. To reduce swelling, apply cold compress to periorbital within the first 48 hours.
7. When sleeping, the patient should keep the head elevated approximately 45°.

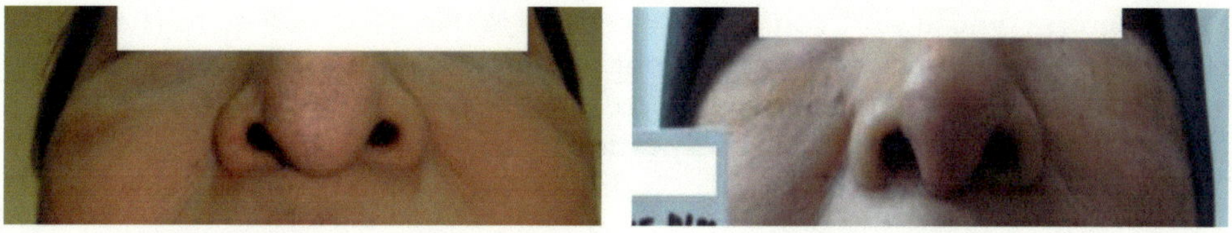

(a) (b)

Figure 10.
Patients with silicone injection usually have wider columella area (a). After the excessive skin of the lateral and the dorsal columella are removed and the implant is placed, the columella area will be more slender, thus shaping a straighter nose (b).

8. If there is a seroma, we can remove it by suctioning using syringe during the follow-up visit.

9. Avoid any trauma for 2 weeks.

10. Remove the stitches on day 10–14.

11. Have a normal diet, but avoid foods that cause excess lip movement such as apples and corn on the cob for 2 weeks after surgery (**Figure 10**).

18. Adjunctive therapy to overcome other complications

The principle of therapy in managing patients with granuloma due to silicone injection is preventing the development of inflammation as it will cause extention of damage.

Evacuation of silicone-induced granuloma should be performed since the liquid silicone in the tissue is persistent and will continuously induce immune response. Although the granuloma has been excised, the remaining silicone, which has migrated to all direction and has been absorbed in the skin, cannot be removed, and therefore, it may cause recurrent granuloma. The remaining inflammation, both granuloma and fibrosis, requires further treatment.

For granuloma or fibrosis that cannot be removed by surgical procedure, other modalities are required to treat the remaining fibrosis and inflammation that can still be seen on the skin, i.e., skin redness and telangiectasia.

19. Fibrosis and remaining granuloma

Some case reports suggest that to treat silicone-induced granuloma, intralesion injection can be used as well as topical treatment of pimecrolimus, which is applied two times daily for 3 months. Topical imiquimod can be used for 8 weeks as well as minoxillin, allopurinol, and oral prednisone at the dose of 30 mg/day [22, 23]. Results of those treatment have not been satisfying although intralesion injection of triamsinolone is more significant for treating the occurring inflammation [24].

Granuloma and remaining fibrosis may also be treated with subdermal injection of triamcinolone acetonide at a dose of 10 mg/ml or a combination of triamcinolone acetonide and 5-fluorouracil. Steroid injection can be performed at the earliest within 2 weeks after wound closure.

The injection is performed once or twice weekly as many as five to seven times. The dose depends on the amount of remaining granuloma and fibrosis, and usually it is at dose of 0.2–0.4 cc per injection.

Etanercept, which works on TNF-α receptor and Fc-IgG1 binding, has been reported providing good result for silicone granuloma [25–27]. The administration of this drug at the dose of 50 mg twice weekly or 25 mg of subcutaneous injection two times a week has offered relatively satisfying results [27].

20. Redness on the nasal skin

When the silicone has entered into the skin, it can cause granuloma due to chronic inflammation. Although the granuloma has been removed, the remaining inflammation, e.g., redness on skin, still exists. One of them is redness due to neovascularization such as telangiectasia due to silicone block in the skin.

Nasal redness and telangiectasia can be reduced using laser treatment. To utilize laser for treatment, we need basic knowledge about the use of laser.

There are three characteristic properties of laser light: monochromatic light. The light contains only a single wavelength, which is determined by the magnitude of released energy. The light has coherent characteristic, and the photon moves regularly as it has the same wavefront to one another.

The light is highly directional. A laser light has a very tight beam that is dense, strong, and concentrated. The three abovementioned characteristics can be achieved since there is a process of stimulated emission.

A light is part of the spectrum of electromagnetic radiation with an energy known as photon, while the molecule that absorbs the light is called chromophore. The energy is transferred from photon entering into chromophore in the skin. After the energy is absorbed, the light can initiate photochemical reaction, heat up the tissue to the state of coagulation or evaporation, and can destroy or detonate tissue structure through extremely rapid localized heating.

Laser is an instrument that produces light beam with certain wavelength or color that is very parallel and coherent. The light wavelength is absorbed maximally by the component of the treated skin. When the absorption characteristics of the target tissue accurately meet the most ideal wavelength, it will develop maximum specificity of laser to tissue interaction.

The mechanism of action of laser is consistent with specific chromophore with certain wavelength. There are three major chromophores in the body, which are hemoglobin, pigment, and water. For redness and telangiectasia cases, we use laser, which mostly works on hemoglobin. The wavelength of laser must be adjusted to the existing problem. Laser light enters the target area on the skin, and subsequently the light is absorbed by specific blood vessel in the skin causing damage on the target blood vessel that contains hemoglobin without injuring the surrounding tissue. We need basic knowledge to perform safer use of laser [28, 29].

In addition to chromophore, we also need to know about thermal relaxation time (TRT). TRT is the time it takes for a target substance to cool half the temperature needed for heating the target without increasing the temperature of surrounding tissue. In order to perform safe procedure, the fluence of a laser pulse must be high enough to heat the target, and the pulse duration must be shorter than the TRT of the target. Each target has its own TRT. For blood vessel, which has TRT up to microseconds, we need long pulse duration; therefore, we should use the long-pulse Nd:Yag laser instead of the QS Nd:Yag laser, which only has pulse duration of nanoseconds. QS Nd:Yag is usually used for tattoo removal.

Laser works based on the selective photothermolysis principle. In this case, it can be used for hemoglobin to treat redness due to the silicone injection. Some lasers that can also be used are vascular laser such as pulse dye laser (PDL) or long-pulse Nd:Yag [30, 31].

A previous study shows that pulse dye laser (PDL) with a wavelength of 595 nm can be used for vascular disorder such as angioma, port-wine stain, rosacea, or other vascular disorders at the dose of 6–8 J/cm^2 every 8 weeks. To prevent side effect, cooling is always performed before laser procedure; some instruments have already had a cryo cooler. The side effects of post-PDL laser treatment are bruising, crust, post-inflammatory hyperpigmentation, particularly for skin types 3–6 according to Fitzpatrick classification [30].

Long-pulse Nd:Yag laser with a wavelength of 1064 nm is also good for treatment of vascular disorder. For deeper vascular disorders and those abnormalities in patients with dark skin types such as the Fitzpatrick skin types 3–6, the instrument will give greater advantages because the 1064 nm wavelength is usually used for pigment chromophore. In contrast, the instrument also has lower safety limit as poor cooling process can often burn the skin. Side effects of long-pulse Nd:Yag laser are bullae, crust, post-inflammatory hyperpigmenta-tion, and scar [31, 32].

In utilizing the long-pulse Nd:Yag laser, we need to set the pulse duration. In silicone-induced disorders, there will be redness on the skin, and one of them is telangiectasia that requires higher dose but lower pulse duration (**Figure 11**).

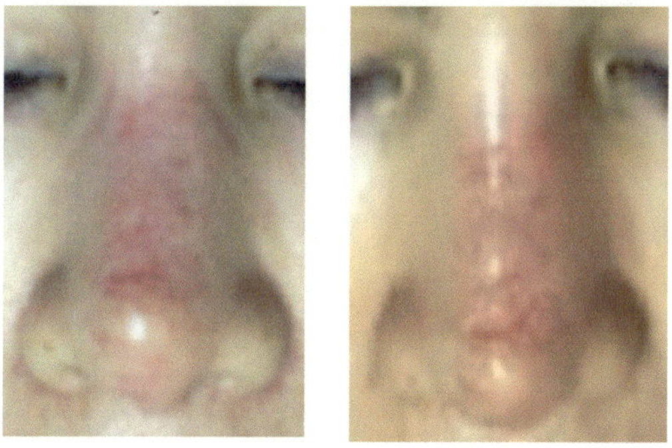

(a) (b)

Figure 11.
Illustration of a patient's skin due to complication of silicone injection on the nasal skin; there is an erythematous skin, and among them, there is a telangiectasia (a). After Nd:Yag laser, the reddish skin and telangiectasia are reduced (b).

In erythematous skin cases, the long-pulse Nd:Yag laser with a wavelength of 1064 nm, at dose of approximately 100 J, spot size of 4, and pulse duration of 10 ms, can be used. For telangiectasia, the power is approximately of 180 J, a spot size of 2, and pulse duration of 5 ms. Sufficient cooling before and after laser procedure should be done, either by using ice pack, air cooling, cryo, or other methods. The laser treatment should be started at a low dose, and the dose is increased gradually for each visit until a change can be observed. The target does not diminish instantly; the color does not always change rapidly; sometimes it only becomes paler.

21. Pitfalls and the management

For a necrotic skin, skin excision on the nasal dorsum is usually done, which is followed by curettage of the surrounding area. We usually clean up the necrotic area and performed wound care, open wound healing enhanced with topical medication that can induce granulation, laser diode, PRP, or others. In general, the wound will heal in 2–3 months.

Excessive granuloma or extensive fibrotic area occurs due to a hard necrotic skin, which creates difficulty in curettage. We can repeat the curettage procedure after a few months, which is followed by steroid injection. For less good-looking nose, excision procedure of the remaining skin can be repeated.

The skin can be burnt due to laser treatment for removing redness or telangiectasia for nasal area. Sufficient cooling before and after laser procedure should be done immediately. Sometime a strong topical steroid such as clobetasol propionate can be applied directly onto the skin after the laser procedure.

22. Conclusion

Treatment for silicone-induced granuloma is not easy because the silicone that enters the skin can migrate and a lot of modalities are required to treat complications. Although the use of silicone injection has been prohibited, we still need to be cautious because there are many cosmetics containing silicone, especially with technological advances that can make the silicone readily absorbed by the skin.

Author details

Ago Harlim
Universitas Kristen Indonesia, Jakarta, Indonesia

*Address all correspondence to: agoharlim@yahoo.com

References

[1] Peters W, Fomarsier V. Complication from injectable material used for breast augmentation. The Canadian Journal of Plastic Surgery. 2009;**17**(3):89-96

[2] Harlim A, Aisah S, Sihombing R. Silicon level in skin tissues of normal female individuals. Journal of Pakistan Association of Dermatologists. 2018;**28**:2

[3] Eighteenth Report of the Joint FAO/WHO Expert Committee on Food Additives, Wld Hlth Org. Techn. Rep. Ser., No. 557. FAO Nutrition Meetings Report Series, No. 54. 1974. Available from: http://www.inchem.org/documents/jecfa/jecmono/v06je42.htm

[4] Liles DT, Lin F. Silicon Elastomeric Particles in Skin Care Applications, Chapter 11. Vol. 1053. Science & Technology Department; 2010. pp. 207-219

[5] Nair A, Jacob S, Al-Dhublab B, Attimarad M, Harsha S. Basic considerations in the dermatokinetics of topical formulations. Brazilian Journal of Pharmaceutical Sciences. 2013;**49**(3):423-434

[6] Alcon Laboratories, Inc. Liquid Silicon Injection. 2010. Available from: http://www.yestheyrefake.net/liquid_silikon_risks.htm [Accessed: August 11, 2010]

[7] Granuloma. Medterms Online Medical Dictionary [Internet]. 1998. Available from: http://medterms.com [Accessed: 20 March, 2011]

[8] James DG, Williams WL. Classification of granulomatous disorders: A clinicopathological synthesis. In: James DG, Zumla A, editors. Granulomatous Disorders. United Kingdom: Cambridge Press; 1999. pp. 17-27

[9] Bondurant S, Ernster V, Herdman R. Antinuclear antibodies and silicone breast implants. In: Safety of Silikon Breast Implants. Washington: The National Academy Press; 1999. pp. 198-214

[10] Lemperle G, Morhenn V, Charrier U. Human histology and persistence of various injectable filler substances for soft tissue augmentation. Aesthetic Plastic Surgery. 2003;**27**: 354-366. DOI: 10.1007/s00266-003-3022-1

[11] Harlim A, Kanoko M, Aisah S. Classification of foreign body reaction due to industrial silicone injection. Dermatologic Surgery. 2018;**9**(44):1174-1182

[12] Price CT, Koval KJ, Langford JR. Silicon: A review of its potential role in the prevention and treatment of postmenopausal osteoporosis. International Journal of Endocrinology. 2013;**2013**:316783

[13] Jugdaohsingh R. Silicon and bone health. The Journal of Nutrition, Health & Aging. 2007;**11**(2):99-110

[14] James DG. A clinicopathological classification of granulomatous disorders. Postgraduate Medical Journal. 2000;**76**(898):457-465

[15] Agustini C, Semenzato G. Biology and immunology of granuloma. In: James DG, Zumla A, editors. Granulomatous Disorders. United Kingdom: Cambridge Press; 1999. pp. 3-16

[16] Granuloma. Dorland's Medical Dictionary [Internet]. Saunders & Elsevier. 2007. Available from: http://www.medical-dictionary.thefreedictionary.com [Accessed: April 13, 2007]

[17] Pollack SV. Wound healing: A review. IV. Systemic medications

affecting wound healing. The Journal of Dermatologic Surgery and Oncology. 1982;**8**:667-672

[18] Adams C, Ratner D. Composite and free cartilage grafting. Dermatologic Clinics. 2005;**23**:129-140, vii

[19] Kovich O, Otley CC. Thrombotic complications related to discontinuation of warfarin and aspirin therapy perioperatively for cutaneous operation. Journal of the American Academy of Dermatology. 2003;**48**:233-237

[20] Sheen JH, Sheen AP. Aesthetic Rhinoplasty. 2nd ed. St Louis: Quality Medical Publishing; 1998

[21] Tardy ME. Rhinoplasty: The Art and the Science. Philadelphia: WB Saunders; 1997

[22] Ellis LZ, Cohen JL, High W. Granulomatous reaction to silicone injection. The Journal of Clinical and Aesthetic Dermatology. 2012;**5**(7):44-47

[23] Arin MJ, Bate J, Krieg T, Hunzelmann N. Silicone granuloma of face treated with minocyline. Journal of the American Academy of Dermatology. 2005;**52**(2):S53-S56

[24] Sharma MD, Hou D, Liu Y, Koni PA, Metz R, Chandler P, et al. Indoleamine 2,3-dioxygenase controls conversion of Foxp3+ Tregs to Th17-like cells in tumor-draining lymph nodes. Blood. 2009;**113**:6102-6111

[25] Pasternack FR, Fox LP, Engler DE. Silicone granulomas treated with etanercept. Archives of Dermatology. 2005;**141**(1):13-15

[26] Desai AM, Browning J, Rosen T. Etanercept therapy for silicone granuloma. Journal of Drugs in Dermatology. 2006;**5**(9):894-896

[27] Styperek A, Bayers S, Beer K. Nonmedical-grade injections of permanent fillers medical and medico-legal considerations. The Journal of Clinical and Aesthetic Dermatology. 2013;**6**(41):20-27

[28] Wheeland RG. Clinical uses of lasers in dermatology. Lasers in Surgery and Medicine. 1995;**16**:2-23

[29] Nelson JS. An introduction to lasers and laser–tissue interactions in dermatology. In: Kaminer MS, Arndt KA, Dover JS, editors. Principles and Practices in Cutaneous Laser Surgery. 1st ed. Philadelphia: Harcourt Saunders; 2002. pp. 59-77

[30] Brauner GJ. Cutaneous laser surgery: Historical perspectives. In: Kaminer MS, Arndt KA, Dover JS, editors. Principles and Practices in Cutaneous Laser Surgery. 1st ed. Philadelphia: Harcourt Saunders; 2002. pp. 3-57

[31] Smit JM, Bauland CG, Winberg DS, Spauwen PHM. Pulsed dye laser treatment, a review of indication and outcomes based on published trials. Journal of Plastic, Reconstructive & Aesthetic Surgery. 2005;**58**(7):981-987

[32] Say Mese E, Gokhan O, Gokemir G. Treatment outcomes of long pulsed Nd:Yag laser for two different subtypes of rosacea. The Journal of Clinical and Aesthetic Dermatology. 2015;**8**(9):16-20

Chapter 2

Costal Cartilage Graft in Asian Rhinoplasty: Surgical Techniques

Sarina Rajbhandari and Chuan-Hsiang Kao

Abstract

Asian rhinoplasty is one of the most difficult and challenging surgeries in facial plastic surgery. As many Asians desire a higher nasal bridge and a refined nasal tip, they undergo various augmentation procedures such as artificial implant grafting and filler injections. Autologous rib graft is a very versatile graft material that can be used to augment the nose, with lesser complications, if done precisely. In this chapter, we have discussed the steps of rib graft harvesting, carving and setting into the nose to form a new dorsal height.

Keywords: rhinoplasty, costal cartilage, Asians, warping

1. Introduction

Asian rhinoplasty is one of the most difficult and challenging surgeries in facial plastic surgery. In Asians, the most common complaints regarding appearance of the nose are a low dorsum and an unrefined tip. Thus, most Asian rhinoplasties include augmentation of the nasal dorsum using either autologous or artificial implant, and/or nasal tip surgery. Clients who have had augmentation rhinoplasty previously frequently opt for revision. Hence, when a client comes for augmentation or Asian rhinoplasty, the surgeon has to confirm whether the client has had any rhinoplasty (or several rhinoplasties) earlier. Artificial nasal implants for augmentation are still in vogue, owing to their simplicity and efficiency, but they are accompanied by several major and minor complications. Revision surgeries for these complications include correcting nasal contour deformities and fix functional problems, and require a considerable amount of cartilage. Revision surgeries are more complex than primary Asian rhinoplasty as they require intricate reconstruction and the framework might be deficient.

The debate regarding optimal graft material still persists. Silastic silicone implants cause a high incidence of early and late complications. There is a modern trend of minimal invasive rhinoplasty, such as threads insertion rhinoplasty and injectable filler rhinoplasty. But, these necessitate repeated procedures which may result in complications.

Autologous cartilage was first used in rhinoplasty in 1900 by Von Mangoldt for syphilitic noses [1]. Septal cartilage, conchal cartilage, and costal cartilage are the most common autologous graft materials used for augmentation. Each of these has their own advantages and disadvantages. Grafts with low resorption rates and sufficient strength for framework support offer consistent long-term results. Since alloplastic material increases the rate of infection, wound contracture and extrusion, autologous tissue is preferred [2].

We need to understand the characteristics of autologous grafts and consider where and how to apply them. Ear cartilage is highly elastic and has sufficient thickness and a natural curve. Hence, it can be used in areas requiring curvature, or can be manipulated by cutting in half and suturing the opposite sides; to be used as a straighter graft [3]. Septal cartilage may be abundant in Westerners but scarce and frail in Asians to be used for augmentation. Furthermore, in revision cases, patients might not have remaining or harvestable septal cartilage or even conchal cartilage. Costal cartilage has an advantage of providing a significant volume, but might cause warping, which is a common and unpredictable complication, and also leaves a scar in the chest [4, 5]. Grafts having low complication rates and high long-term patient satisfaction are considered ideal for grafting [6]. These qualities are noticed in autografts and are regarded as better alternatives for Asian rhinoplasty. Every Asian patient undergoing rhinoplasty must be properly evaluated as the outcome may vary in every patient.

In this chapter, we have discussed our techniques of harvesting and using the costal cartilage to augment and enhance the nose in Asians. Despite its abundance, costal cartilage also brings complications. But, when autologous rib cartilage rhinoplasty is performed by an experienced surgeon, it will provide an excellent, reliable, and lasting result with low risk [7]. Below, we have mentioned how to minimize the complications of harvesting and utilizing a costal cartilage and improve our surgical results.

2. Preoperative assessment

An elaborate understanding of the client's expectations should be understood. What the surgeon might feel as an appropriate nasal dorsum height or nasal tip projection might not be satisfactory for the client. In these instances, simulation techniques to exhibit the probable post operative outcomes can be discussed with the client, but realistic results should be clarified.

Before surgery, we ask the client to carry out common investigations required for general anesthesia; such as complete blood count, bleeding profile, blood grouping, renal function tests, X-ray of the chest and electrocardiogram. Rib harvesting might also call for a CT scan of the chest to check for ossification of the rib, which is often seen in individuals over 40 years of age, although, we have experienced circumstances where even younger individuals presented with ossified ribs.

The surgery can be carried out by a single team or could be a two team approach where one team works on the nose and the other focuses on harvesting the rib. The second approach accounts for a lesser operative time and the rib is generally harvested from the left side, since the surgeon operating on the nose is usually on the right. In our practice, we have the same team operating on the nose and harvesting the rib, hence, we harvest the rib from the right chest wall.

3. Harvesting the rib cartilage

The incision site is normally over the right sixth or seventh rib. Some surgeons also prefer the floating rib at the inferolateral costal margin [8]. Similarly, when additional cartilage is required, we also harvest the eighth or ninth rib. The medial portion of the seventh rib cartilage is long enough for a caudal septal extension graft or a columellar strut and a dorsal implant can be easily carved from its midrib portion, which is wide and thick enough. A premaxillary graft can be carved from its lateral portion. Our incision is a short linear inframammary incision. The incision site scar is the most major concern while harvesting a rib, but a smaller incision with detailed suturing and hiding the scar in the inframammary fold conceal the post operative scar and settle the client's issues regarding it. After infiltrating local anesthesia, we make an incision with a No. 10 or 15 blade, at the middle of the inframammary fold, around 2–3 cm in length, although in beginners, it is better to make a longer incision for better view and ease. In males, the incision is made directly over the concerned rib. To avoid exaggerated scarring, it is better to not extend the incision beyond the vertical line from medial nipple-areola-complex [9]. When a female client has decided to have a breast augmentation in the future, we make sure to place out incision 7.5–8 cm below the nipple, which is generally the anticipated new inframammary fold. In a female who has already undergone breast augmentation, we have to be careful to not rupture the capsule of the implant.

We then perform meticulous dissection along the subcutaneous tissue and muscle fascia plane, reaching and dividing the extracostal muscle directly over the rib. The oblique abdominis and rectus abdominis muscle are vertically split and retracted. The underlying rib is identified and checked for ossification by pricking it with a syringe needle. Medially, our dissection is the junction of the rib cartilage with the sternum and laterally is the osteochondral junction. The selected rib is thus exposed, followed by a longitudinal incision through its perichondrium, along the length of its central axis. Careful circumferential subperichondrial dissection is carried out underneath the rib, exposing its posterior aspect. One must be cautious to not injure the perichondrium, which might cause complications such as pneumothorax. From the superior aspect of the rib, we also harvest some perichondrium to use as graft material. Under direct vision, a curved or right angled elevator is used to lift the rib from the underlying perichondrium. The rib is incised halfway through its thickness with a knife and proceeded with an elevator. Medially, the rib is incised at its attachment near the sternum and laterally, at the bony rib junction. This harvested rib measures 4.5–6 cm in length (**Figure 1**). In revision cases, we may require to harvest a part of the adjacent rib as well. These graft materials are submerged in normal saline with gentamicin solution. While operating on the nose, the graft remains in this solution and is observed for warping.

Before closure, we irrigate the donor site with thermal saline and check for absence of air bubbles when positive pressure ventilation is provided. This will help us ensure that there is no injury to the lung pleura/or absence of pneumothorax. Closure is done in layers. To reduce post operative pain and to facilitate proper drainage of blood, the fascia over the muscle is closed with interrupted sutures, using vicryl 3-0 sutures. Subcutaneous closure is done by vicryl 4-0 sutures and skin closure by nylon

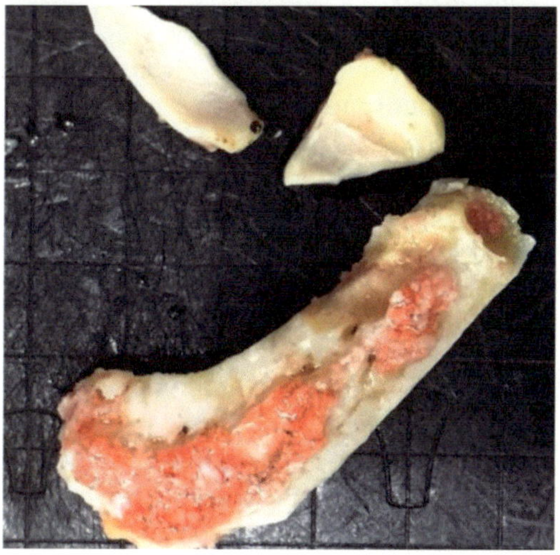

Figure 1.
Perichondrium is harvested along with the 7th rib cartilage. The cymba and cavum concha are also harvested.

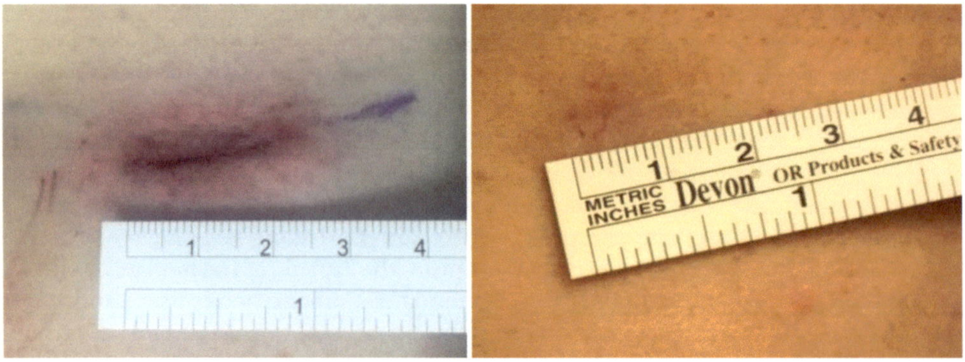

Figure 2.
The scar immediately after wound closure is almost invisible 1 year after surgery.

6-0 interrupted sutures. 5-0 PDS or vicryl may be used subcutaneously to avoid suture removal (**Figure 2**).

4. Dissection of the nose

We make an inverted V incision along the midcolumella, which is connected with bilateral marginal incisions. The skin flap is elevated to the level of perichondrium of the lower lateral cartilage. We use tenotomy scissors and elevators for this step. In presence of excess subcutaneous tissue in thick skin clients, it may be removed (but not aggressively) for more post operative tip definition. Septum is approached by separating the two medial crura and the subperichondrial plane of the caudal septum is identified. The septum is exposed by elevating bilateral mucoperichondrial flaps and separated from the upper lateral cartilage. A dorsal-caudal L-shaped strut of the septum is preserved for septal support. This harvested septal graft may be used as caudal septal extension graft (CSEG) or splint grafts, but they may be deficient in revision cases.

5. Harvesting the conchal cartilage

Cavum and cymba conchal cartilage is preferred for tip grafts and lateral crura strut grafts (LCSG) due to its curvature and elasticity. This is done via a post auricular approach, making an incision with a no. 15 blade. Skin and perichondrium are elevated from the underlying perichondrium and dissection is proceeded using appropriate scissors or also blunt dissection can be done with cotton-tip applicators. We should stop the dissection short of the cartilage of the external auditory canal. We generally preserve the radix helicis, to preserve the ear position. The cymba and cavum conchal are harvested as two separate entities and put in the saline-gentamicin solution along with the harvested rib and septum. The incision is sutured using nylon 6-0 running mattress sutures.

6. Carving the rib cartilage

Before carving the costal cartilage graft, we measure the height of the nose at the nasion, rhinion and nasal tip. This helps us to decide the extent of carving of our graft. The dorsal graft and spreader grafts are carved from the middle portion of the harvested rib. The client's skin thickness is kept in consideration while carving the graft. In thick skinned people, the final outcome may not be as obvious as in thin skinned people. Sharp lines and angles appear blunted under a thick skin (**Figure 3**).

We carve the graft into a "fusiform" shape; which is tapered off at both ends with a wider mid region (**Figure 4**). The concave portion of the graft acts as the bottom of the implant. Precise carving and smoothening, with serial checking by inserting the graft inside the nasal skin-soft tissue flap is done, to determine the suitable height and width of the anticipated nasal shape. Balanced cuts are made in the cartilage in several directions to prevent warping. Most warping occurs within 15–60 min of harvesting and it is important to wait for early warping and reshape the graft before placement [10, 11]. Thus, the graft is carved equally on both sides, maintaining a balanced cross section of the graft.

The superior aspect of the graft to be placed over the radix is placed in an uphill converging manner to rest over the underlying bone (**Figure 5**). An additional rib cartilage may be assembled underneath the onlay graft for extended augmentation.

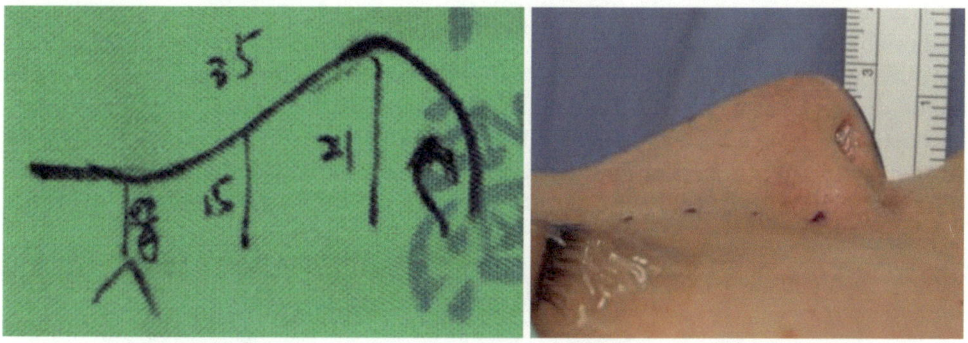

Figure 3.
Measurement of the nose is taken at the nasion, rhinion and nasal tip to determine the pre operative and post operative differences.

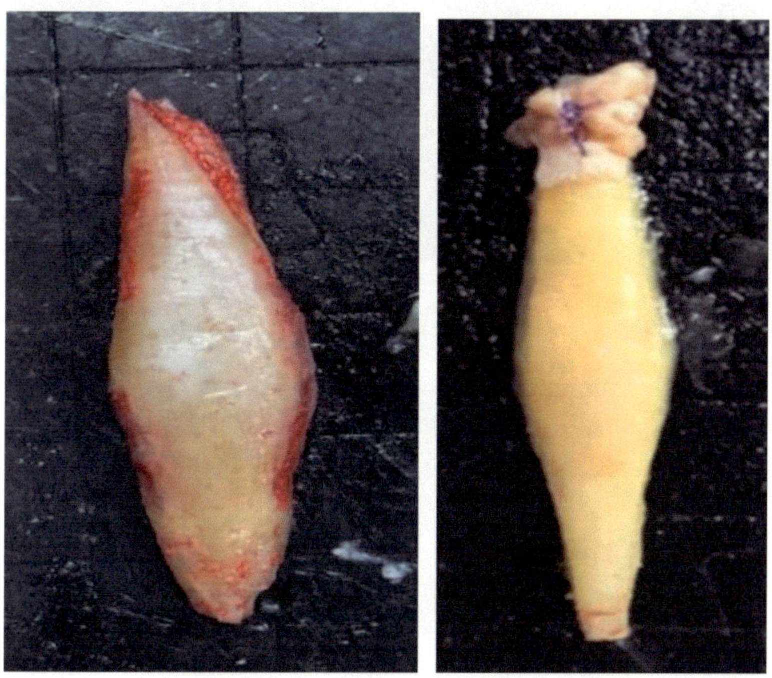

(a) (b)

Figure 4.
(a) Rib graft is carved in a fusiform shape. (b) Perichondrium is sutured to the cephalic end of the graft to augment the radix height.

The caudal end of the harvested rib graft is tapered and it should stop right above the lower lateral cartilages, for mobility of the lower one third of the nose. The final result should be a nose that is in tone with the rest of the Asian facial features. The onlay graft is secured in position by fixing with 2 or 3 fixation sutures with PDS 5.0, around the graft and through bilateral upper lateral cartilages. Capsule from a previous silicone implant is preserved during nasal dissection and used as a camouflage graft. Similarly, the harvested perichondrium from the rib or temporalis fascia can also be used to wrap around the rib and hide irregularities (**Figure 6**).

From the remaining portions of the rib, splint grafts, lateral crura strut grafts, caudal septal extension grafts (CSEG), columellar struts, etc. are carved (**Figure** 7). A CSEG is approximately 2 mm in thickness and trapezoidal in shape. If the septal cartilage is sufficient, a CSEG may be carved from the harvested septal cartilage. It can be fixed to the nasal L-strut in an end to end or overlapping fashion. Splint grafts are used on either side of the CSEG/L-strut complex to preserve the strength and resilience of the lower third of the nose. Extensive osteotomy may require spreader grafts as well to prevent internal valve collapse. In our experience, we have concluded that Asian clients rarely require osteotomies. Intranasal medial and lateral osteotomies are done for crooked bony dorsum. Medial osteotomy is done from the beginning of junction of upper lateral cartilage and nasal bone at a paramedian position; it is gently curved outwards at an angle of 10–15° as it proceeds upwards

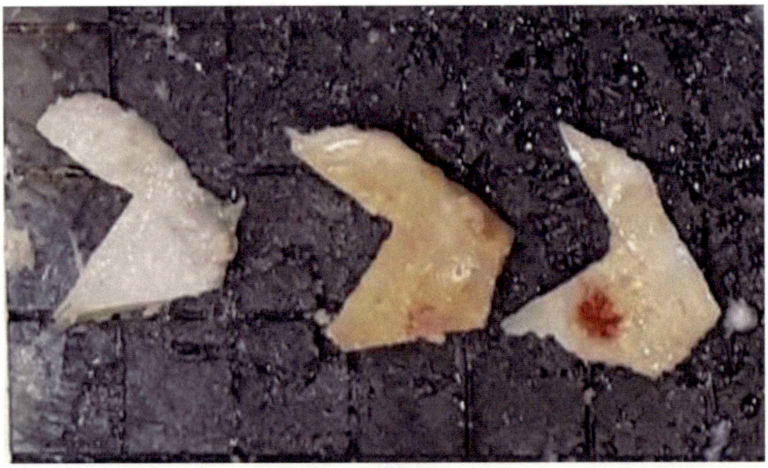

Figure 5.
CSEG and splint grafts carved from the remaining portion of the harvested rib.

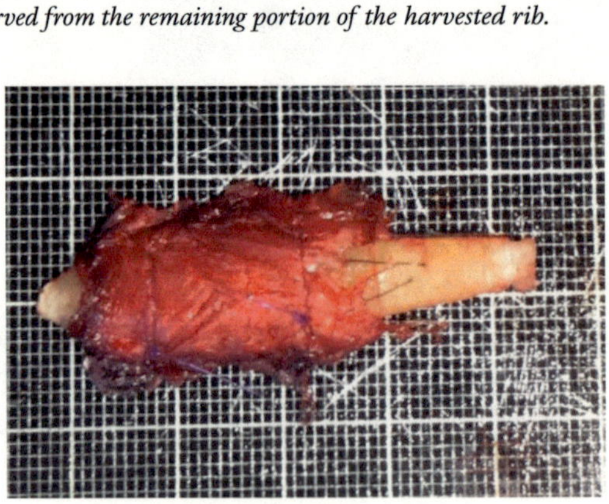

Figure 6.
Deep temporal fascia wrapped around the graft to hide irregularities.

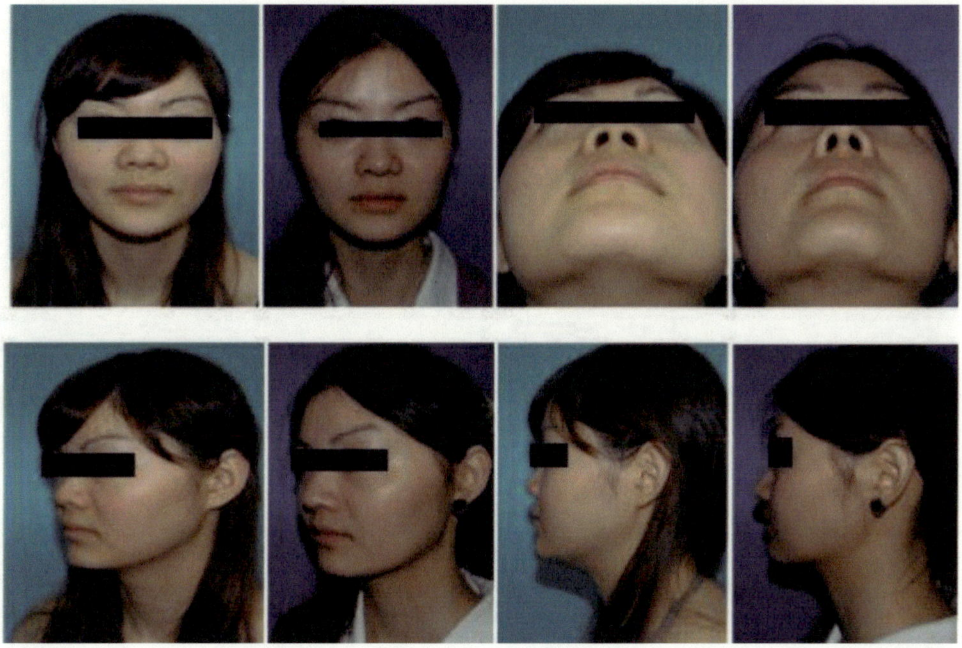

Figure 7.
Case 1. A young female underwent open rhinoplasty with autologous rib cartilage augmentation. The pictures are taken before and 1 year after surgery.

to connect with the lateral osteotomy. Lateral osteotomy is started just above the level of the inferior turbinate and is usually performed in a low-low-high fashion in Asians.

When augmentation is done, the client might not need an alar flare reduction afterwards, but in some cases, it may be performed.

7. Discussion

Artificial nasal implants (silicone, goretex) and filler injections have widely been used to augment the dorsum, increase the length of the nose and project the nasal tip in Asians. However, these render complications of their own such as a shrunken nose, an artificial appearance and hard feel of the nose, skin discoloration, and migration of implants, skin erosion and extrusion [12]. Asians expect a facially harmonized look and thus undergo more than three revision surgeries, to correct previous surgeries, improper use of implants, or surgical complications [13]. Rib graft is an ideal material for primary or revision rhinoplasty, owing to its abundant supply and rigid support (**Figures 8–10**). Chances of skin infection, necrosis and shrinkage are less with the use of costal cartilage. Many surgeons prefer harvesting the rib from the sixth, seventh or occasionally the eighth rib [14]. In female clients, the sixth costal cartilage is preferred as the oblique incision scar to harvest it may be hidden in the inframammary fold, and females generally would not prefer a long nose. In males, we harvest the seventh rib for a longer dorsum. Some Asian clients seek a Western esthetic nose; hence, surgeons may need to harvest more than one rib. The most common complications of rib grafting are the chances of warping and infection. Precise carving as mentioned above and soaking the rib in saline-gentamicin solution may reduce the risk of post surgery warping. Meticulous dissection during surgery, effective antibiotics and postoperative care are important. Multiple grafts may affect skin tension, and scar tissues from previous surgeries can reduce the vascular supply to the graft and increase probability of infection [15].

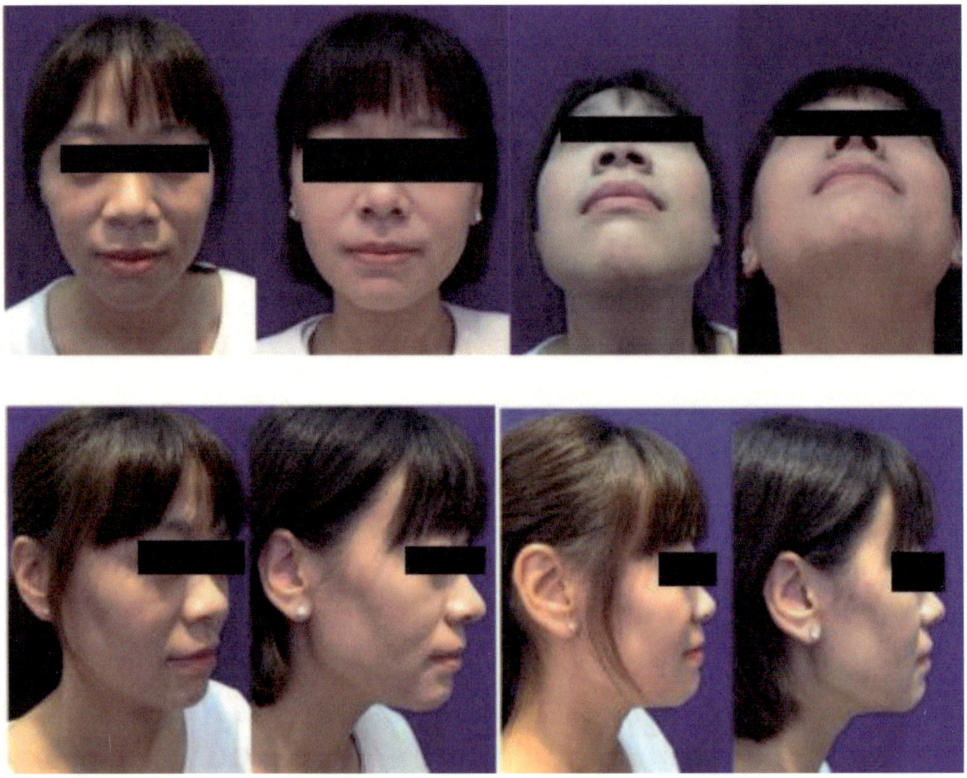

Figure 8.
Case 2. This female underwent open rhinoplasty with autogenous costal cartilage grafting and ear cartilage grafting for tip refinement. These pictures are taken before and 3 months after surgery.

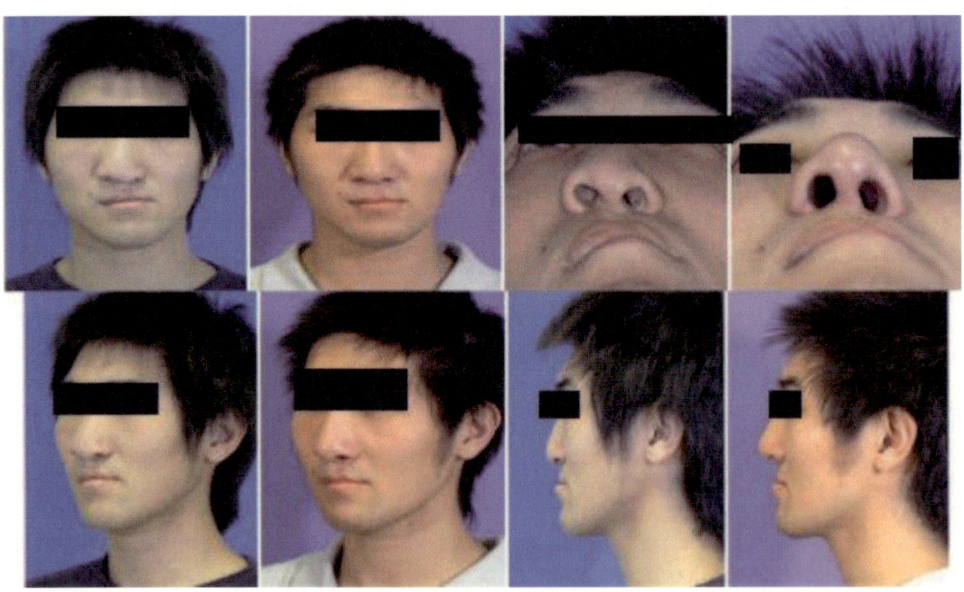

Figure 9.
Case 3. A case of cleft nasal deformity underwent open rhinoplasty with autologous rib cartilage grafting. These pictures are before and 1 year after surgery.

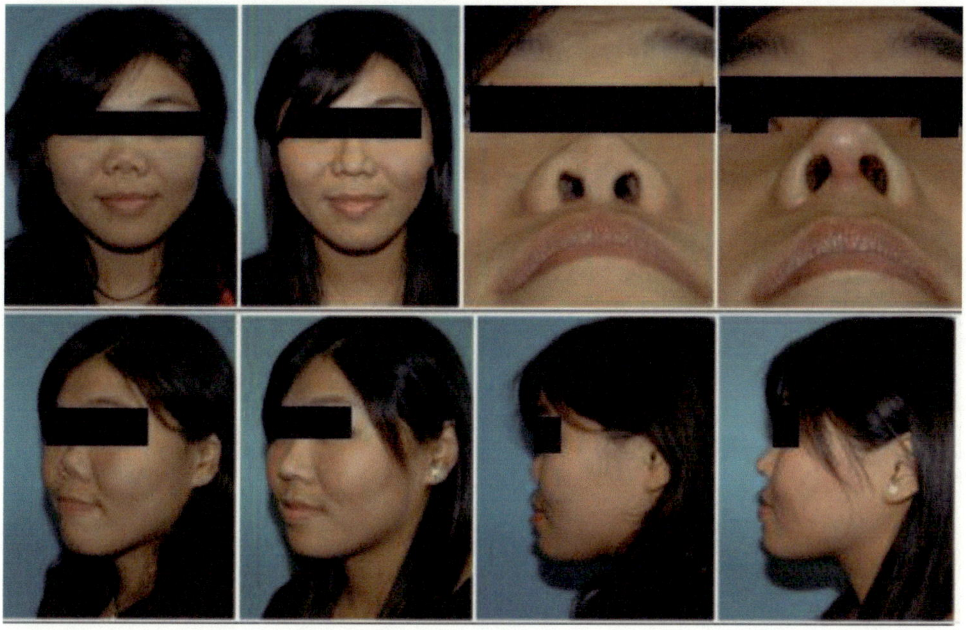

Figure 10.
Case 4. A case of saddle nose deformity who had augmentation with silicone implant previously. Two ribs were harvested for nasal dorsal, premaxillary and paranasal augmentation.

Cadaver rib may also be used for rhinoplasty, but since it is not live, autologous tissue, it may form a capsule due to unassimilated tissue, has higher long term absorption rate, risk of transmitting diseases such as HIV, hepatitis, etc. and possibility of soft tissue loss if infection control is delayed [16, 17]. Calvarial bone grafts are also becoming popular with the advances in craniofacial surgery. When morphologically compared with endochondral bone, membranous bone has a thicker cortical plate, smaller endocortical cancellous area, and stronger intracortical struts [18]. Hence, calvarial bones are also a good material of choice for augmentation rhinoplasty. This bone also resembles the other facial bones and can be easily incorporated into the nasal framework. The risk of significant absorption is less, however, there is a possibility of injury to the dura and intracranial structures, hematoma/seroma, with inadequate training [19].

The fundamental strength of the osseocartilaginous rib graft lies in replacing like with like [8]. A rib graft allows for bony integration with the nasal dorsum, immobilizes the graft and allows for meticulous sculpting of the nasal tip. However, autologous costal cartilage should be used keeping the possibility of complications in mind, especially when a large amount of graft material is required.

Conflicts of interest

There are no conflicts of interest.

Authors' contributions

Dr. Chuan-Hsiang Kao made contribution to the conception and design of the study and provided cases and material for the study.

Dr. Sarina Rajbhandari made contribution to the presentation of the text and concept of the study.

Declarations

None to be made.

Financial support and sponsorship

None.

Author details

Sarina Rajbhandari[1] and Chuan-Hsiang Kao[2]*

1 Department of Otolaryngology-Head and Neck Surgery, Starr Hospital, Kathmandu, Nepal

2 Department of Otolaryngology-Head and Neck Surgery, Tri-Service General Hospital, Taipei, Taiwan

*Address all correspondence to: chuanhsiang@yahoo.com.tw

References

[1] Lupo G. The history of aesthetic rhinoplasty: Special emphasis on the saddle nose. Aesthetic Plastic Surgery. 1997;**21**(5):309-327

[2] Marin VP, Landecker A, Gunter JP. Harvesting rib cartilage grafts for secondary rhinoplasty. Plastic and Reconstructive Surgery. 2008;**121**:1442-1448

[3] Endo T, Nakayama Y, Ito Y. Augmentation rhinoplasty: Observations on 1200 cases. Plastic and Reconstructive Surgery. 1991;**87**(1):54-59

[4] Jang YJ, Alfanta EM. Rhinoplasty in the Asian nose. Facial Plastic Surgery Clinics of North America. 2014;**22**(3):357-377

[5] Sajjadian A, Rubinstein R, Naghshineh N. Current status of grafts and implants in rhinoplasty: Part I. Autologous grafts. Plastic and Reconstructive Surgery. 2010;**125**(2):40e-49e

[6] Kao CH, Hsu CH, Lee JC, Wang HW, Tsai KK. Customized material choice for Asian rhinoplasty: How we do it. Clinical Otolaryngology. 2011;**36**:165-170

[7] Toriumi DM, Pero CD. Asian rhinoplasty. Clinics in Plastic Surgery. 2010;**37**:335-352

[8] Christophel JJ, Hilger PA. Osseocartilagenous rib graft rhinoplasty. Archives of Facial Plastic Surgery. 2011;**13**(2):78-83

[9] Tebbetts JB. The inframammary approach for augmentation. In: Augmentation Mammoplasty. St. Louis, MO: Mosby; 2010. pp. 251-288

[10] Adams WP, Rohrich RJ, Gunter JP, et al. The rate of warping in irradiated and nonirradiated homograft rib cartilage: A controlled comparison and clinical implications. Plastic and Reconstructive Surgery. 1999;**103**:265-270

[11] Cakmak O, Ergin T. The versatile autogenous costal cartilage graft in septorhinoplasty. Archives of Facial Plastic Surgery. 2002;**4**:172-176

[12] Lam SM. Revision rhinoplasty for the Asian nose. Facial Plastic Surgery. 2008;**24**(3):372-377

[13] Suh MK, Ahn ES, Kim HR, Dhong ES. A 2-year follow-up of irradiated homologous costal cartilage used as a septal extension graft for the correction of contracted nose in Asians. Annals of Plastic Surgery. 2013;**71**(1):45-49

[14] Gunter JP, Cochran CS. Dorsal augmentation with autogenous rib cartilage. Seminars in Plastic Surgery. 2008;**22**:74-89

[15] Holt GR, Garner ET, McLarey D. Postoperative sequelae and complications of rhinoplasty. Otolaryngologic Clinics of North America. 1987;**20**:853-876

[16] Song HM, Lee BJ, Jang YJ. Processed costal cartilage homograft in rhinoplasty: The Asian medical center experience. Archives of Otolaryngology–Head & Neck Surgery. 2008;**134**(5):485-489

[17] Welling DB, Maves MD, Schuller DE, Bardach J. Irradiated homologous cartilage grafts. Long-term results. Archives of Otolaryngology–Head & Neck Surgery. 1988;**114**(3):291-295

[18] Hardesty RA, Marsh JL. Craniofacial onlay bone grafting: A prospective

evaluation of graft morphology, orientation, and embryonic origin. Plastic and Reconstructive Surgery. 1990;**85**:5-14

[19] Cheney ML, Gliklich RE. The use of calvarial bone in nasal reconstruction. Archives of Otolaryngology–Head & Neck Surgery. 1995;**121**:643-648

Chapter 3

Botulinum Toxin for the Face

Amin Amer, Mohamed Amer and Hagar Nofal

Abstract

Botulinum toxin is a corner stone in the facial esthetics. It has been used for decades for various medical and esthetic indications. Botulinum toxin is a neurotoxin that interferes with the transmission at the neuromuscular/neurosecretory junctions by inhibiting the release of acetylcholine. An in depth knowledge of the functional anatomy of facial muscles is required to obtain the best results of the botulinum toxin injections. In this book chapter, a detailed practical guide for the FDA approved and the off label uses of botulinum toxin in the face is presented. The recently developed new indications are listed. The lengthy experience with botulinum toxin injections has proved safety and tolerability of the procedure; however, the probable complications, and steps for their prevention and management are highlighted.

Keywords: Botulinum toxin, facial esthetics, Crow's feet, anti-aging, forehead lines

Botulinum toxin (BTXN) is an exotoxin produced by the anaerobic, Gram positive, spore forming bacteria; *Clostridium botulinum.* There are seven serotypes A-G. A and B serotypes are the ones currently used commercially. The toxin is 150 kDa polypeptide, formed of heavy chain and light chain bound by heat sensitive disulfide bonds and noncovalent forces. The toxin may be formulated in a simple - free from proteins - form e.g. incobotulinum or complexed with proteins as hemagglutinin and "nontoxic molecule" to form onabotulinum toxin and abobotulinum toxin [1, 2]. It is essential to keep in mind that the different types of the toxin are not similar in their biological effects and potencies [1]. The currently available formulations are unique, so their doses are not interchangeable, and the dose response curves are probably not parallel [3].

1. Mechanism of action

It inhibits the release of acetylcholine (ACh) from nerve endings via cleavage of SNARE protein complex responsible for ACh release. Thus it affects the presynaptic nerve endings at the neuromuscular junction (NMJ) causing muscle paralysis (main site of action) [1], and the cholinergic postganglionic autonomic nerve fibers innervating the eccrine, salivary and tear exocrine glands (neurosecretory junction) [2, 4]. This inhibition is reversible within variable periods of time via the regeneration of synaptic junctions [1, 4].

Indications:

Despite being widely used for multiple indications, botulinum toxin's FDA approved indications are limited **Table 1**.

The indications of BTXN in the face is summarized in **Table 2**.

IntechOpen

	Forehead lines/ Cosmetic	Other^
Onabotulinumtoxin (Botox)	Yes	Cervical dystonia, severe primary axillary hyperhidrosis, strabismus, blepharospasm
Abobotulinumtoxin (Dysport)	Yes	Cervical dystonia, blepharospasm
Incobotulinumtoxin (Xeomin)	Yes	Cervical dystonia, blepharospasm
Rimabotulinumtoxin #(Myobloc)	No	Cervical dystonia, blepharospasm

^Upper limb spasticity, chronic migraine, overactive bladder and urinary incontinence.

Table 1.
FDA approved indications of botulinum toxin.

Indications	Responsible muscles	Unites and Technique
Upper Face		
Glabella lines (**Figure 1**)	**Procerus** **Corrugator** supercilii Depressor supercilii Orbicularis oculi	**Procerus:** Intramuscular, single injection point, perpendicular to the skin, 2–4 U [3] **Corrugator:** Intramuscular 1–3 injection points at each side, First injection point 0.5–1 cm above the medial orbital rim, 2nd injection point 1 cm above and lateral to 1st injection point, 2–4 U/ point [3]
Lateral canthal lines (Crow's feet) (**Figure 2**)	**Orbicularis** oculi	Intradermal or SC injection of the lateral muscle fibers, 3 injection points 1–2 cm lateral to the orbital rim, 2–5 U/ point, total dose is 6–15 U [3, 5].
Forehead Lines[1] (**Figure 3**)	**Frontalis**	The target is to only soften, not to completely eliminate, forehead lines; the patient ideally can still elevate the eyebrows to a lesser extent than prior to treatment [1, 3, 6]. Intramuscular or intradermal (especially near eyebrow), 4–8 injection points in 1–2 rows, start injection with the upper lateral fibers to the mid forehead inferiorly (stop 2 cm above the brow), 2–4 U/point, total 8–25 U [6]. For narrow forehead less injection points and lower doses are used. To maintain neutral brow position and arch the corrugator supercilii, procerus and superiolateral fibers of orbicularis oculi are treated at the same time or a few days before frontalis injection [1, 3].
Bunny lines (Nasal oblique lines)	**Nasalis (upper fibers)**	Intramuscular, 2–3 injection points, 2 U/point [3].
Gummy smile[2]	**Levator labii superioris alaeque nasi**	Intramuscular (at the site of levator labii superioris alaeque nasi and zygomaticus minor convergence with the insertion of levator labii superioris, 1–2 injection points, 0.5–2 U/ point [3]
Lower Face		
Perioral rhytides (smokers' lines)	**Orbicularis oris**	BTXN injection is recommended for deep rhytides, superficial ones need either resurfacing or hyaluronic fillers Intradermal, 2–5 injection points, 0.5–1 U/ point [3, 6].
Marionette lines	**Depressor anguli oris**	Intramuscular, 1–2 points/ side, 2–3 U/ injection point. The main injection point is the posterior aspect of the depressor anguli oris muscle at the superior margin of the mandible, and at least 1 cm lateral to the oral commissure [3, 6].

Indications	Responsible muscles	Unites and Technique
Mentalis overactivity	**Mentalis muscle**	Intramuscular, 1–4 injection points 3–5 U/ point.
Masseter overactivity (square jaw) / bruxism	**Masseter muscle**	Intramuscular, 1–6 injection points/ side, 5–15 U/injection. Average of 3 points are injected at the center of the masseter square at least 1.5 cm from the mandibular border [7], one superiorly and 2 inferior and laterally. Caucasians tends to need lower doses than Asians with longer periods of effect. The injection is to be directed at the posterolateral corner [6, 8, 9].
Platysmal bands	**Platysma**	Only for patients with obvious platysmal bands, and good cervical skin elasticity with no or minimal submental fat [6]. Intramuscular or deep intracutaneous, typically 2 bands are injected at a time with 3 points of injection in each band, 1–1.5 cm apart, 1–5 U/ injection point, total 15 U/ band and 30 U/ session [3, 6]. For horizontal neck folds: Superficial intradermal, 1–2 U/ point equidistantly in the folds.
Facial asymmetry Caused by Bell's palsy		The contralateral active side is injected using small doses (1–2 U) of Ona BTXN into muscles of the normally functioning side (the zygomaticus, risorius and orbicularis oris muscles) and 5–10 U into the masseter muscle [6, 10]. For post Bell's palsy synkinesis the paralyzed side is injected either as four periocular injections or into the affected muscles as orbicularis oculi, orbicularis oris and frontalis using the total dose of 10–40 units [10, 11].
Acne and Sebum production		Excess sebum production: Few reports of BTXN use as intradermal (1 cm apart forehead and check) or intramuscular injection (five fixed points in the forehead) in the forehead for management of excess sebum production 2 U/injection site [12]. Acne: one clinical trial has been registered using 1.5–3 U/ active lesions. The trial has been terminated with no published reports on the results [13]
Gustatory sweating (Frey syndrome)		Intracutaneous injections of 4 U /cm^2 [14]

Muscles written in bold *are the injected muscles. Facial musculature varies between males and females, with increased strength and bulk in men. Thus, higher doses and increased number of injection points are generally required in men in all regions of the face [5].*
[1]*Brow position is lowered with age "brow ptosis". Glabellar complex injection (20–40 U) lead to immediate lateral eyebrow elevation, followed by an entire brow lift that peaked 12 weeks post treatment. This effect is due to the toxin diffusion into the lower medial frontalis muscle fibers with subsequent increased tone in the upper and lateral frontalis fibers. Forehead lines is recommended to be done simultaneously with brow lift to maintain a neutral position for the eye brow [6].*
[2]*Exposure of ≥2 mm of the gingiva on smiling [8]. Done for younger patients with strong lip elevator complex [6].*
[3]*Youthful face is a heart shape with fullness in the upper part and tapering toward the mandible [1]. It is essential to exclude parotid gland hypertrophy either primary or secondary to pathology as Sjögren syndrome or bulimia nervosa or parotid gland mass using clinical assessment and CT imaging, or volume loss related masseteric prominence [3, 15].*

Table 2.
Botulinum toxin neuromuscular indications in the face.

2. Storage and reconstitution

The various BTXN products are supplied as lyophilized powder containing vials except for rimabotulinumtoxin which is supplied in a liquid form [1].

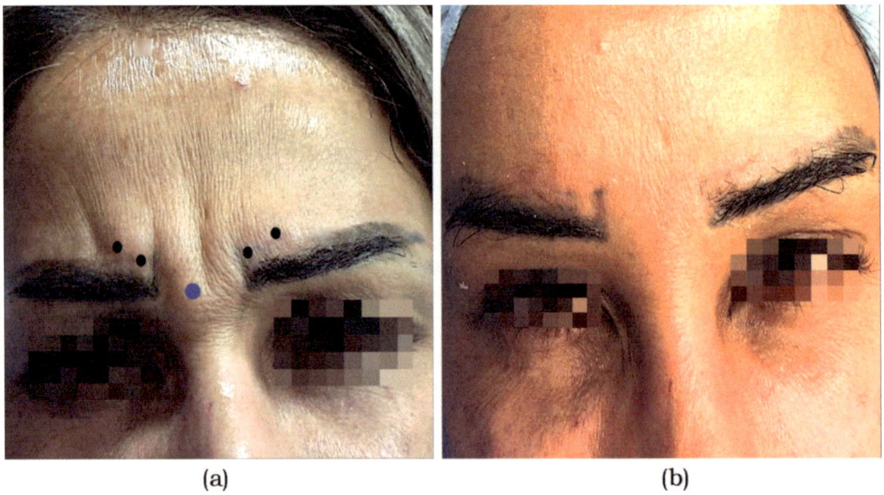

Figure 1.
Glabellar complex injection. (a) before: ***Procerus*** *(blue dot) single intramuscular perpendicular to the skin, 2–4 U,* ***corrugators*** *(black dots)***:** *2 intramuscular injection points 2–4 U/point; first injection point 0.5–1 cm above the medial orbital rim, 2nd injection point 1 cm above and lateral to 1st injection point. (b) after.*

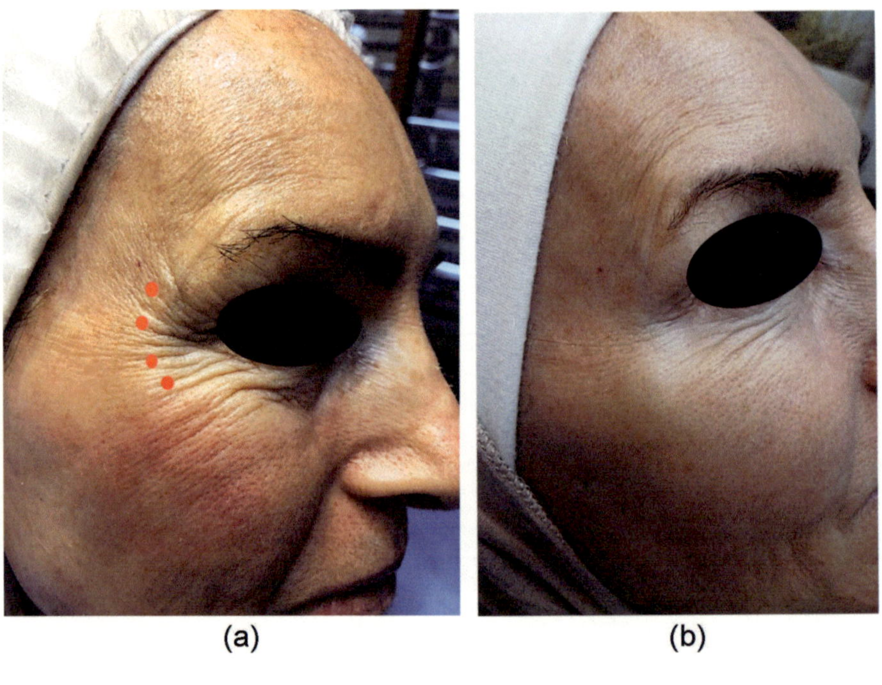

Figure 2.
Lateral Canthal lines injections. (a) before: 3 intradermal injection points 1–2 cm lateral to the orbital rim 2–5 U/ point. (b) After.

To reconstitute the powdered BTXN, a non- preserved saline, preserved (bacteriostatic) saline or lidocaine can be used as a diluent agent, the laters are associated with less pain on injection [1, 4].

The reconstituted vial can be used for up to 4 weeks safely if kept frozen at – 20°C or refrigerated at 4°C [1, 4].

A single vial can be used for multiple patients, as long as there is safe and sterile reconstitution and injection techniques are followed [1, 16].

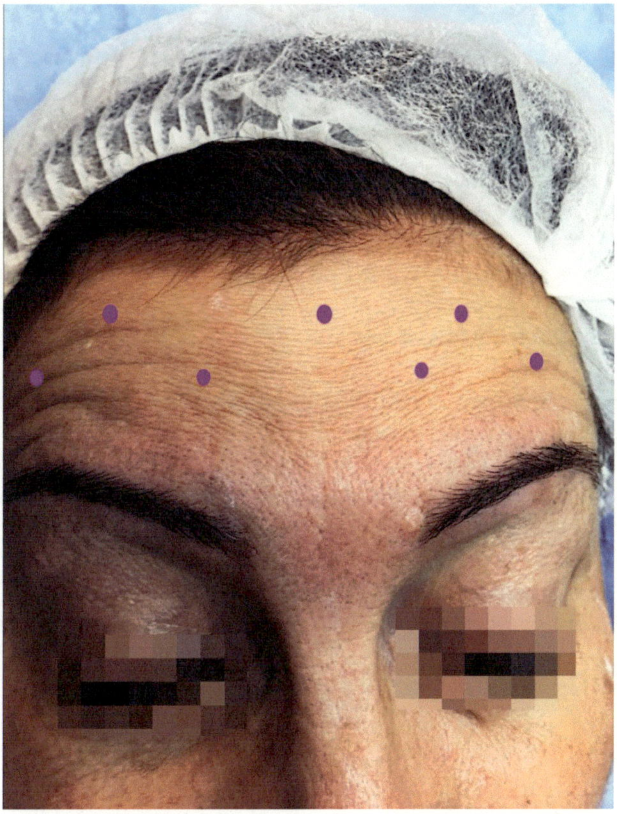

Figure 3.
Forehead lines injection. 4–8 intramuscular - intradermal near eyebrow - injection points in 2 rows, starting with the upper lateral fibers (stop 2 cm above the brow), 2–4 U/point.

There are variable methods for BTXN reconstitution. 100 U vial of onabotuliunum A is commonly reconstituted in 2 cc of the diluent, which means there is 5 U/ 0.1 cc. 500 U of abobotulinum toxin A is diluted in 2.5 cc of the diluent so that there is 20 U/0.1 cc [7].

3. Clinical considerations

3.1 Pretreatment assessment

The key to successful intervention is tailoring the treatment plan to every patient's need and combining different procedures to achieve best outcome [3]. Combination with hyaluronic acid fillers is increasingly utilized to optimize outcomes. The combined treatment with fillers can be considered for all regions, including the upper face [16].

For esthetic indications, the current trend accepted by both patients and physicians is to use BTXN in the least effective dose, injection points, and at longer intervals to achieve muscle activity modulation rather than muscle paralysis [3].

Assessment of the muscles should be performed at rest and at maximum muscle contraction [5].

Muscular and bony landmarks are to be used to identify the injection points [3].

It is recommended to discuss with the patients the black box warning and to document consent [8].

3.2 Pretreatment preparation

1. Removal of makeup

2. Thorough skin cleansing using 70% alcohol before, during, and after injection

3. Topical anesthesia can be used to minimize the pain.

4. Sterile injection technique using 1 ml 30 gauge needle.

3.3 Post treatment instructions and care

1. Ask the patient to frown and smile repeatedly for 30 minutes following injection to minimize the diffusion outside the injected muscles.

2. Avoid massaging the treated areas within 3 hours after injection to minimize diffusion to other non-injected muscles

3. For upper face, avoid bending over or strenuous physical activity (controversial), lying down or sleeping for 3 hours following the injections.

Contraindication [8, 17]:

1. Infection at site of injection.

2. Known hypersensitivity reaction to any of the ingredients (toxin or human albumin).

3. Preexisting inflammatory skin condition at site of injection e.g. acne, contact dermatitis, atopic dermatitis and psoriasis.

4. Pregnancy (reports of premature delivery no causal relationship was proven) or lactation, it is categorized as C drug

5. Neuromuscular disease or patients with preexisting difficulties in swallowing or breathing e.g. myathenia gravis, amyotrophic lateral sclerosis and myopathies. Those patients are more predisposed for marked muscle weakness, dysphagia or respiratory compromise the toxin unmasked subclinical disease in some patients, however BTXN injection was used successfully in others.

6. Co-administration with drugs interfering with neuromuscular activity as aminoglycosides, lincosamides, cholinesterase inhibitors, curare-like depolarizing blockers, succinylcholine, magnesium sulfate, calcium channel blockers, quinidine, and polymyxin.

7. Anti coagulant therapy or bleeding disorders.

4. Complications

Neurotoxins treatments are proven to be remarkably safe. All the reported adverse events are related to injection techniques, dosage, or volume of injection. Allergic reactions are very rarely encountered.

General	
	How to avoid
Pain	Topical anesthetics, lidocaine for vial reconstitution, small gauge (30–32) needles and ice packs.
Edema/ Erythema	Ice packs application immediately before and after injection.
Ecchymosis	Avoid the superficial vasculature (proper lightening and stretch the skin for better visualization) Patient counseling regarding the need to stop NSAIDs, aspirin or anticoagulant therapy prior to injection for ≤1 week.
Headache	Those at risk can receive prophylaxis acetaminophen.
Neutralizing antibodies	They block the pharmacologic activity of the treatment affecting 0.3–6% of patients, its incidence is much higher in patients receiving toxin treatments for medical indications. BTXN-B products are more immunogenic than BTXN-A. It is controversial whether there is cross reactivity across different serotypes of the toxin, however it is worth trying to shift the patient to another serotype e.g. from BTXN-A to BTXN-B as a solution for neutralizing antibodies.
Procedure specific	
Glabellar complex	**Eyelid ptosis** due to toxin diffusion through the orbital septum, paralyzing the levator palpebrae superioris muscle, specially when injecting the mid pupillary line 1 cm above the bony supraorbital rim to obtain horizontal brow. Avoided by the lateral corrugator muscle subdermal injection and do not inject within a 1-cm distance above the superior orbital rim. It is treated with α-adrenergic eye drops, such as apraclonidine or phenylephrine eye drops.
Frontalis	• **Brow ptosis** due to overtreatment of the frontalis muscle. Avoided by keeping the lower most injection points 1.5 cm above the brow. • Excessive lateral brow elevation **"Quizzical" brows** due to central fibers treatment, while the lateral fibers inadequately treated causing lateral brow elevation.
Crow's feet	• **Ectropion**, **diplopia**, or **lateral lower eyelid drooping** due to injection of the lateral rectus muscle so avoid deep intramuscular injection within 1 cm from the lateral bony orbit • **Upper lip ptosis** due to injection into zygomaticus muscle. This can be avoided by not injecting during smiling and do not follow the lines inferiorly.
Masseter hypertrophy	• Salivary gland enlargement • **Smile limitation** and/or **asymmetry** which is avoided by injecting into the square-shaped safe area that is bounded by a line joining the oral commissure to the ipsilateral earlobe superiorly, the mandibular border inferiorly and the anterior and posterior borders of the muscle identified while patient grinds on his/her teeth.
Platysma	**Dysphagia, hoarseness, weakness** of the flexors of the neck, **dry mouth**. This is avoided by keeping the injection units ≤50 U

Conflict of interest

None.

Author details

Amin Amer*, Mohamed Amer and Hagar Nofal*
Dermatology Department, Faculty of Medicine, Zagazig University, Zagazig, Egypt

*Address all correspondence to: aminamer74@gmail.com
and hnofal@medicine.zu.edu.eg

References

[1] Giordano CN, Matarasso SL, Ozog DM. Injectable and topical neurotoxins in dermatology: Basic science, anatomy, and therapeutic agents. J Am Acad Dermatol. 2017 Jun 1;76(6):1013-1024.

[2] Trindade de Almeida AR, Montagner S. Botulinum Toxin for Axillary Hyperhidrosis. Hyperhidrosis. 2014 Oct 1;32(4):495-504.

[3] Sundaram H, Signorini M, Liew S, Trindade de Almeida AR, Wu Y, Vieira Braz A, et al. Global Aesthetics Consensus: Botulinum Toxin Type A--Evidence-Based Review, Emerging Concepts, and Consensus Recommendations for Aesthetic Use, Including Updates on Complications. Plast Reconstr Surg. 2016 Mar;137(3):518e–529e.

[4] Nawrocki S, Cha J. Botulinum toxin: Pharmacology and injectable administration for the treatment of primary hyperhidrosis. J Am Acad Dermatol [Internet]. [cited 2020 Feb 7]; Available from: https://doi.org/10.1016/j.jaad.2019.11.042

[5] Lowe NJ. Aesthetic Uses of Botulinum Toxins. In: Rook's Textbook of Dermatology, Ninth Edition [Internet]. Ninth Edition. Wiley-Blackwell; 2016. Available from: https://onlinelibrary.wiley.com/doi/abs/10.1002/9781118441213.rtd0036

[6] Carruthers A, Carruthers J, Trindade de Almeida A. Botulinum Toxin. In: Dermatology: 4th Edition. 4th Edition. New York: ELSEVIER; 2017.

[7] Kwon K-H, Shin KS, Yeon SH, Kwon DG. Application of botulinum toxin in maxillofacial field: part I. Bruxism and square jaw. Maxillofac Plast Reconstr Surg. 2019 Oct 1;41(1):38-38.

[8] Giordano CN, Matarasso SL, Ozog DM. Injectable and topical neurotoxins in dermatology: Indications, adverse events, and controversies. J Am Acad Dermatol. 2017 Jun 1;76(6):1027-1042.

[9] Klein FH de M de S, Brenner FM, Sato MS, Robert FMBR, Helmer KA. Lower facial remodeling with botulinum toxin type A for the treatment of masseter hypertrophy. An Bras Dermatol. 2014;89(6):878-884.

[10] Cooper L, Lui M, Nduka C. Botulinum toxin treatment for facial palsy: A systematic review. J Plast Reconstr Aesthet Surg. 2017 Jun 1;70(6):833-841.

[11] Monini S, De Carlo A, Biagini M, Buffoni A, Volpini L, Lazzarino AI, et al. Combined protocol for treatment of secondary effects from facial nerve palsy. Acta Otolaryngol (Stockh). 2011 Aug 1;131(8):882-886.

[12] Shuo L, Ting Y, KeLun W, Rui Z, Rui Z, Hang W. Efficacy and possible mechanisms of botulinum toxin treatment of oily skin. J Cosmet Dermatol. 2019 Apr 1;18(2):451-457.

[13] Dayan SH. Double-Blind, Randomized, Placebo-Controlled Study to Determine the Safety and the Efficacy of Using Botulinum Neurotoxin Type A Injections for Subjects With Mild to Moderate Acne Vulgaris [Internet]. clinicaltrials.gov; 2018 May [cited 2020 Jun 4]. Report No.: NCT00765375. Available from: https://clinicaltrials.gov/ct2/show/NCT00765375

[14] Freni F, Gazia F, Stagno d'Alcontres F, Galletti B, Galletti F. Use of botulinum toxin in Frey's syndrome. Clin Case Rep. 2019 Jan 31;7(3):482-485.

[15] Bae GY, Yune YM, Seo K, Hwang SI. Botulinum Toxin Injection for Salivary Gland Enlargement Evaluated Using Computed Tomographic Volumetry.

Dermatol Surg [Internet]. 2013;39(9). Available from: https://journals.lww.com/dermatologicsurgery/Fulltext/2013/09000/Botulinum_Toxin_Injection_for_Salivary_Gland.22.aspx

[16] Alam M, Tung R. Injection technique in neurotoxins and fillers: Indications, products, and outcomes. J Am Acad Dermatol. 2018 Sep 1;79(3):423-435.

[17] Carruthers A, Kiene K, Carruthers J. Botulinum A exotoxin use in clinical dermatology. J Am Acad Dermatol. 1996 May 1;34(5, Part 1):788-797.

Chapter 4

Combining Helium Plasma-Driven Radiofrequency with Nanofat for Contouring

Diane Irvine Duncan

Abstract

Many energy sources have been utilized to optimize tissue behavior following traditional liposuction. Peer-reviewed data to date show that radiofrequency has been shown to cause more skin and soft tissue contraction than other energy sources. While external RF can improve skin quality and create new collagen formation, tissue contouring has not been successful with topical energy application. However, the use of subdermal RF has been utilized to generate directional shaping and contouring in addition to skin tightening. An understanding of the way soft tissue contracts over time as collagen fibers develop is based on both the science of soft tissue energy response and experience in treating large numbers of patients. The Apyx Renuvion device is 510(k) cleared for soft tissue coagulation. In most cases of facial and body contouring, the ability to add volume in specific regions is as important as the skill to remove it. Since some liposuction is commonly performed as a part of the Renuvion contouring process, frequently this lipoaspirate is used to augment focal depressions or areas of soft tissue atrophy. The recent development of mechanical processing of macrofat into smaller particles, as well as nanofat, has widened the scope of the use of adipose-derived tissue.

Keywords: radiofrequency, plasma, nanofat, minimally invasive, neck, facial contouring

1. Introduction

Radiofrequency-assisted liposuction (RFAL) has been performed since 2008 [1]. Early devices were used to heat tissue prior to lipoaspiration, and the early cannulas performed both tissue heating and liposuction. Users gradually changed the order of the steps in the procedure, as it became clear that removing some of the adipose insulation prior to heating enhanced soft tissue contraction. Original versions of cannulas contained heating elements in a bipolar configuration that are allowed for treatment at multiple depths. A new, smaller version of radiofrequency was introduced in 2014. This device was monopolar and utilized a 10 or 15 cm wand-like cannula that was placed under the skin. Best suited for smaller areas, the device was capable of targeted nerve ablation as well as soft tissue coagulation. Both devices are considered "bulk heaters" as the subcutaneous cannula tip heats the soft tissue in gradients, hotter near the cannula tip and cooler away from the device tip [2]. The mechanism of action was the coagulation of the lax stromal collagen fibers, which resulted in overlying skin contraction as an indirect effect. In 2016, a helium plasma-driven radiofrequency device created for laparoscopic cutting and coagulation was used externally for skin resurfacing. An esthetic surgeon then placed the device under the skin, causing soft tissue coagulation and subsequent skin tightening in this region. Instead of targeting a large area of soft tissue, this device emits very small multidirectional pulses of RF energy that are impedance driven. The energy is delivered in a fractional manner. All subdermal RF devices cause mild soft tissue contraction initially, followed by gradual ingrowth of a new stromal collagen scaffold over time in the treated region. Safety is optimized with the helium plasma device, as the external skin temperature rarely reaches 39 degrees C. The treatment target is the fibroseptal stroma, not the overlying dermis.

Nanofat has been used for many purposes including enrichment of traditional fat grafts, in combination with myostimulation, and intradermal injection in patients who desire skin resurfacing without epidermal ablation. While the FDA considers nanofat or SVF produced with collagenase a drug, mechanical instead of chemical tissue manipulation does not fall into the "drug" or maximally manipulated category [3]. Mechanical devices must obtain a 510(k) clearance and are single use only. However, the individual devices cost quite a bit less per use than a tissue processing laboratory within the operating room would. Examples of nanofat processing units include the Nanocube (Lipocube, London) and Tulip devices (Tulip Medical, San Diego, CA). Nanofat is created from fatty lipoaspirate, and the cells that remain are fragile, prone to death when desiccated or roughly handled. The solution can be combined with particulate fat in order to enhance the quality of fat grafts. It can be injected intramuscularly following myostimulation. Nanofat can be injected into regions with radiation damage in order to lessen the deterioration of the skin and soft tissue. Also injected directly into the skin, nanofat can improve the quality of aging skin by stimulating dermal fibroblasts. It is not recommended to apply nanofat topically as very few cells will survive in this environment.

While either procedure alone has benefit, the combination of helium plasma-driven RF to treat soft tissue for localized volume reduction plus nanofat-enriched grafts for focal volumetric enhancement corrects most deformities in the subdermal region. The addition of intradermal nanofat injection helps to enhance the appearance of aging skin without creating any superficial injury.

2. Background

Initially, the purpose of adding radiofrequency energy to traditional liposuction was to prevent the inevitable postoperative skin laxity in cases of moderate to large volume reduction. The Vectra measurement of skin surface area contraction [4] showed 26% surface area reduction at 6 weeks posttreatment and 36% at 1 year. Corresponding measurements of skin contraction obtained with mechanical stimulation after SAL showed contraction of 10% at 6 weeks and only 8% at 1 year. While laser-assisted liposuction did tighten the skin surface area more effectively than SAL at 13–17% measured skin tightening [5, 6], none of the other energy assists generated significant measured associated skin tightening. As patient expectations continue to grow, these also drive both technical and clinical development. Demands for a smooth, taut contour following treatment have encouraged surgeons to adopt techniques that will result in better outcomes than were common a decade ago. Changes that have been noted during this development phase include lower power settings, fewer passes—but passes at multiple depths—and more contouring in regions that need more attention. As with other energy-based devices, the RFAL procedure has evolved from a basic company guideline of three to five passes per region to more of a sculpting approach. Because most surgeons also perform excisional techniques, the ability to visualize which region needs 33% skin contraction or less is a good guideline for treatment. If there is a localized region with extreme pendulosity, skin excision might be recommended. In order to transition from simple skin tightening to directional shaping, both vision and experience help to guide the practitioner in the therapeutic application of RF energy.

The popularity of using nanofat has grown rapidly over the past several years. With FDA-cleared devices for mechanical production of progenitor cells, the process has become affordable for most physicians and patients. Nanocube TM has been cleared for mechanical adipose tissue processing. This device produces millifat, microfat, and nanofat. The harvested macrofat is serially transferred through a cutting screen. The cube is rotated between ports 1 and 2 to produce millifat. Microfat is produced following several passes through the screen between ports 2 and 3. Nanofat production requires passage of the adipose tissue through ports 3 and 4. There is an average of between 50,000 and 70,000 MSCs in each cc of this particular nanofat, though no adipocytes remain.

3. Materials and methods

The Apyx Renuvion device has recently obtained a 510(k) clearance for a new handpiece that is significantly smaller in diameter than the original footprint (**Figure 1**). A bullet nose contour at the tip aids in a precise placement, and the two-side firing ports achieve a 360-degree directional energy placement. The handpieces are slightly flexible for ease of use in curved regions. As the energy is emitted just proximal to the handpiece tip, end hits are prevented. At a 3 mm diameter, instead of the previous 5 mm, the device can now be introduced through a small port created with a 16-gauge needle. Erythema and mechanical abrasion at the access port are reduced due to a graduated indicator system near the handpiece tip, warning the user that the device tip is near. More access points can now be placed without

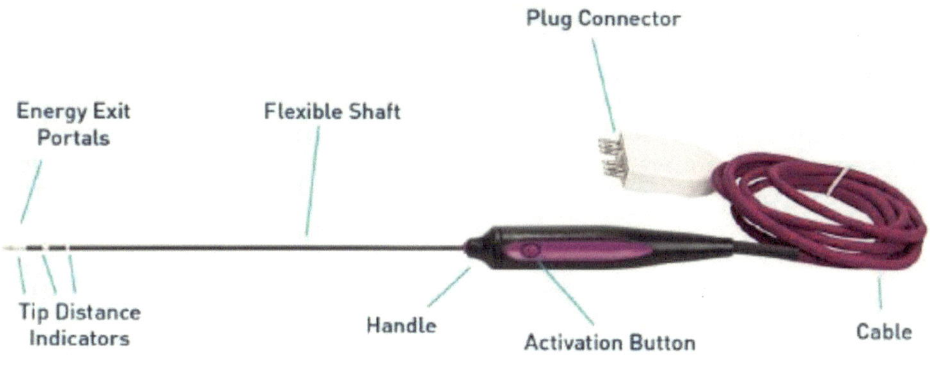

Figure 1.
New handpiece is approved by the FDA for soft tissue coagulation: side port configuration of tip—testing demonstrated that the first locations of highest external tissue temperatures were treatment transition areas (i.e., transitions from treated tissue to untreated areas) when energy was delivered distally from tip of the device. Based on the results of this testing, the APR handpiece was designed to have plasma discharged radially from the side ports of the tip as opposed to distally; indicator lines on tip of device—the second location where the external tissue temperatures were the highest was areas within approximately 40 mm from the incision site providing access to the subdermal plane. There is a risk of this area being overtreated since the treatment strokes of the device converge at the incision site. In order to prevent overtreatment of this area, indicator lines were included on the shaft of the Renuvion APR device to provide awareness to the user that the tip is nearing the incision site. The user is also instructed to stop activation of the device when the indicator line becomes visible at the incision site; and epidermal marking templates—provided in device packaging as a mean for the user to mark 40 mm from the incision site on the patient. This will prevent possible overtreatment where treatment passes converge at the incision site.

concern for pronged visible erythema. Also, more regions can be easily treated with the redesigned handpiece. The lower face, arms including the elbows, knees, and ankles are excellent targets for HPDRF treatment. There is no requirement for liposuction; soft tissue contraction in such areas as the neck, breast, arms, knees, and axilla can be performed following tumescent infusion.

Optimal settings range from 60 to 80% power and 1.5 to 3 L/min helium flow rate. While a minimum of three passes per region is recommended for the average treatment region, thin areas such as the nonfatty neck, upper arms, decollette, and knees should be treated with no more than two passes per region in order to avoid postoperative fibrosis.

While general anesthesia reduces the need for large volumes of tumescent fluid infusion, small areas can be treated under local anesthesia. Patients may find that the inhalation of nitrous oxide can reduce perceived discomfort during tumescent infusion. The limitations of local/ tumescent anesthesia include possible lidocaine toxicity and increased sensitivity to discomfort when the second region is being treated.

Following sterile prep and draping, access ports that were pre-marked in the upright position are injected with local anesthetic. A small 20-gauge infusion cannula is used to infuse standard Klein's solution into the treatment region at multiple levels. The recommended fluid ratio is 1:1, meaning that approximately 1 cc of lipoaspirate is planned for each cc of tumescent infused. Because helium plasma RF is impedance driven, too little fluid creates a high-resistance field, while too much fluid does not allow the tissues to heat optimally. Liposuction is performed prior to RF heating in cases where it is indicated. If no liposuction is performed, pre-tunneling with a 3 mm cannula is recommended in order to establish the proper planes prior to application of RF energy. It is strongly recommended that at least three communicating access ports be created, so that helium gas is allowed to escape. Postoperative crepitus can be reduced by aspirating from each access port following RF heating. Three to five passes are recommended in each treatment region if the area is moderately lipodystrophic. In patients with very thick fat layers, up to eight passes can be performed at multiple varying depths. It is possible to create a seroma if depths are not varied. If energy is applied only superficially, the lax adipose layer will not reattach to the underlying fascia, and an optimal correction will not be achieved. It is important not to scrape the underside of the skin in an effort to achieve skin contraction. This can cause linear depressions that are very difficult to correct. Recommendations to stay at least 5 mm under the base of the dermis will improve the possibility of a smooth skin surface postoperatively. When performing a secondary case, marking of any preoperative depressions in the standing position is ideal. Following any revisional liposuction of the protruding areas, any treatment with RF heating

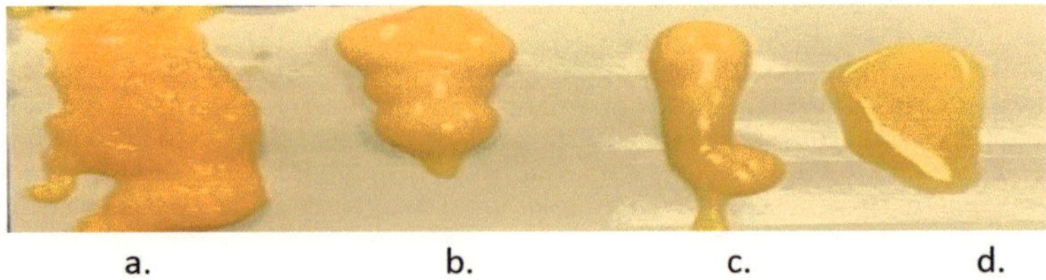

Figure 2.
(a) Macrofat: Best for structural repair and contains stroma and fat >2 mm particle size. (b) Millifat: Obtained with first pass through Nanocube. 2 mm particle size. (c) Microfat: Obtained with second pass through Nanocube. Able to inject into the dermis. (d) Nanofat: This solution has progenitor cells but no adipose and can inject intradermally with a 30-gauge needle.

should remain at the Scarpa's fascia or below in order to avoid creating more superficial fibrosis. After the use of RF heat, fat grafting should be performed with slight overcorrection in the depressed regions. Specific regional contouring descriptions are given below.

Nanofat was processed following the harvest of fat using traditional liposuction techniques with negative pressure of only 10 mm Hg. In order to reduce extravasated free fatty acid contents, filtration rather than centrifugation was used for initial fat processing. Macrofat (particles measuring >3 mm) was then processed in the Nanocube in order to produce millifat, microfat, and nanofat (**Figure 2**). Macrofat was injected in regions needing more structure, such as the bra roll depression, chin, and the prejowl sulcus. Millifat was injected in the infraorbital hollows in order to avoid lumpiness. Microfat can be injected with a 25-gauge needle and is used for supporting the deep dermis or for mixing with biostimulatory agents such as hydroxyapatite.

Nanofat can be combined with all types of particulate fat and also can be injected by itself with a 30-gauge needle. The stimulation of dermal fibroblasts is the primary purpose with superficial nanofat injection.

4. Results

The combination of using helium-driven plasma in the subcutaneous space for contouring has been enhanced with the development of a new handpiece. Ease of use, especially in areas with thin skin, striae, and small surface areas, has made the operative procedure more straightforward. Due to the slightly flexible nature of the cannula, directional shaping in regions such as the jawline, neck, lateral breast and axilla, upper arm, and knees has become possible.

The use of Renuvion is no longer limited to skin surface area contraction, though this use is off-label. The ability to shape soft tissue is difficult, even with traditional surgical techniques. If the fibroseptal network can be manipulated in such a way that a new form with defined shape is possible without skin excision, the stage is set for optimized outcomes.

The addition of fat grafting in certain regions also enhances results. For example, many women have skin pendulosity as well as localized lipodystrophy in the bra roll region. Frequently, there is an associated depression, due to the tethering of the dermis to the midlevel Scarpa's fascia. By releasing the tether and creating a superficial subdermal tunnel that is then filled with transferred fat, the deformity can be fully corrected without surgical skin excision (**Figure 3**).

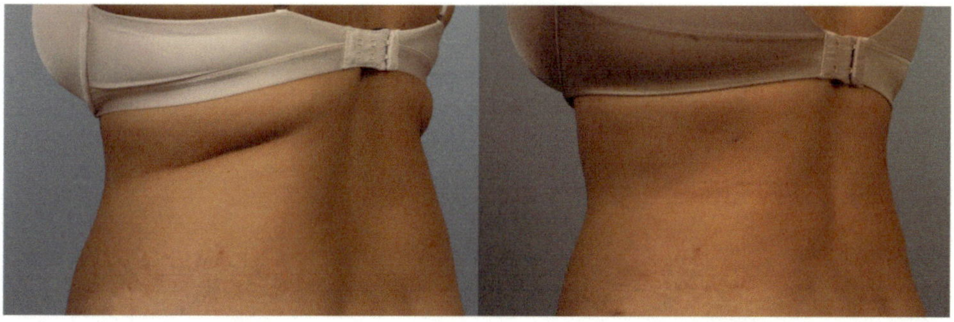

(a) (b)

Figure 3.
(a) 38-year-old before surgery. (b) 3 months post-Renuvion treatment of bra roll and flanks.

Other areas that benefit from this combination are the lower face and jawline. A common problem with aging is bony resorption of the maxilla and mandible. This process causes visible jowling due to skin and stromal laxity as well as hollowing of the prejowl sulcus and gonial notch. The process of soft tissue aging is characterized by gradual loss of the scaffold, or fibroseptal network, in the fatty layer (**Figure 4**). The use of radiofrequency energy in the multiple levels of adipose stroma will regenerate this framework over the period of 1 year.

Hollow regions tend to be focal instead of diffuse. Known regions of accelerated aging include the prejowl sulcus, gonial notch, oral commissures, distal nasolabial folds, and medial infraorbital regions. Temporal hollowing, also known as the "old horse" phenomenon, also creates an aged appearance even in younger patients. By restoring the smooth and full contour of the face and jawline, apparent age reduction can be accomplished with a process known as microlifting [7].

A third novel use of combined RF energy plus nanofat-enriched grafting is in male body contouring. Formerly reserved for liposuction plus etching [8], the addition of myostimulation plus fat transfer to the male contouring armamentarium has broadened the scope of male body contouring. By combining electromagnetic energy [9] with stem cell tissue enrichment, muscle volume can be enhanced in ways not achievable in the gym. **Figure 5** shows results of a man treated 2 years ago with Renuvion and his 2-year result.

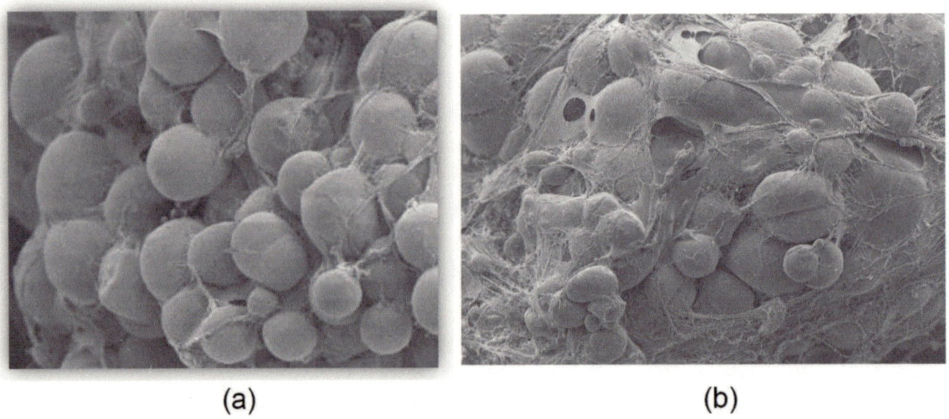

Figure 4.
(a) SEM of aging adipose tissue. Note the lack of collagen support network. (b) 3 months post-RF treatment of the adipose layer; the collagen binding network is restored.

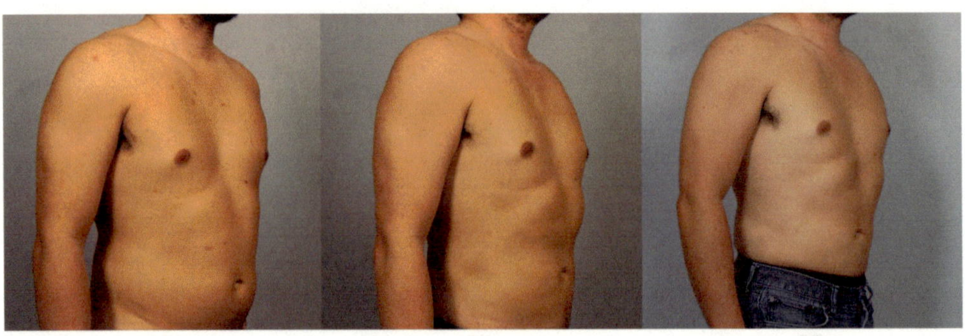

Figure 5.
(a) 38-year-old before surgery. (b) Early result 6 weeks post-op. (c) Result at 2 years post-op.

Myostimulation with radiofrequency energy combined with nanofat injection can also enhance the small muscles of the face. As we age, the combination of bone atrophy, muscle thinning and atrophy, and soft tissue volume loss [10] can lead to the development of a negative facial expression [11]. The combination of RF myostimulation at subcoagulative levels combined with intramuscular injection of progenitor cells can result in shortening of the long, attenuated upper lip by 3 mm or more without a "bullhorn" skin excision (**Figure 6**). The addition of erbium laser resurfacing can definitively optimize the long-term outcome in patients ≥60 years of age. In patients with mild to moderate neck laxity, the use of plasma-driven radiofrequency in the neck and submental region can be an alternative to a surgical neck lift, even with patients over 60 (**Figure 7**).

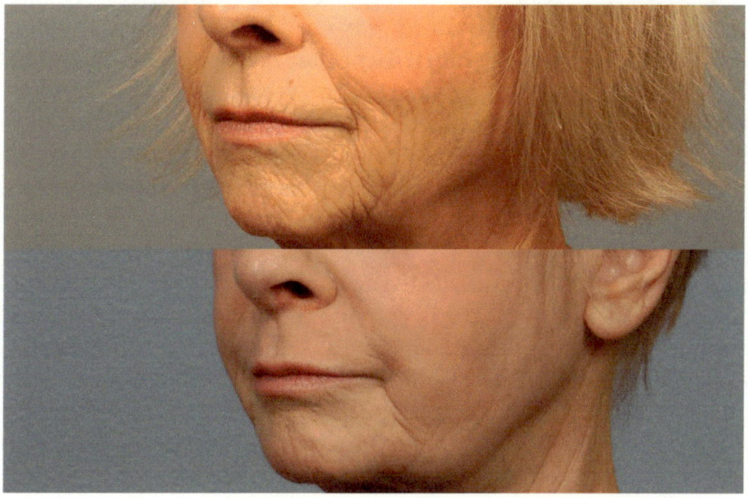

Figure 6.
(Above) 73-year-old woman before surgery. (Below) 6 months post-laser resurfacing, fat grafting, and RF myostimulation to the upper lip.

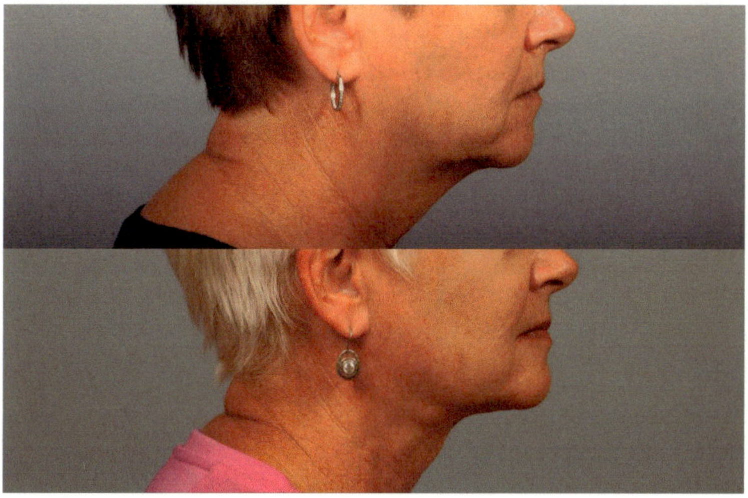

Figure 7.
(Above) 61-year-old before treatment. (Below) Same patient 3 months post-Renuvion-assisted neck lift. No skin was excised.

5. Discussion

Regenerative medicine is rapidly gaining a large market share of the esthetic market [12]. The procedures that utilize the patient's own tissues make sense to most people, and the ability to generate a prolonged improvement without significant temporary deformity or downtime resonates with potential customers. As the popularity of minimally invasive or noninvasive procedures soars [13], esthetic practices are enthusiastically seeking solutions that are safe and effective. By understanding the causes of apparent aging as well as minimally or noninvasive options for skin and soft tissue restoration, esthetic practitioners are able to address these concerns in ways that patients identify with. The optimal combination of electromagnetic and RF energy plus nanofat-enriched fat transfer can optimize long-term outcomes of rejuvenative procedures.

The use of subdermal RF energy can restore the framework or scaffold that supports the overlying skin. With commonly used liposuction techniques, especially superficial liposuction, the integrity of that framework can be compromised, and a cannula defect or localized depression can result. Even with subdermal radiofrequency devices, if the cannula is used to scrape the underside of the dermis, interrupting the subdermal fibroseptal network, the adjacent soft tissue contraction will paradoxically amplify the defect as the soft tissue near the injury contracts. A uniform network of contractile hypodermis is needed for a smooth postoperative surface.

The combination of subcutaneous tissue contraction and stabilization and regeneration of the overlying skin will provide the optimal outcome in most facial and body contouring efforts. If underlying muscle laxity is a contributing factor to the deformity, electromagnetic stimulation of the affected muscle is recommended. Restoration of the stromal/skin complex's attachment to the underlying fascia can be achieved by applying RF energy at the junction of these two layers. **Figure 8** shows a patient treated with plasma-driven RF in the abdominal region. Treatment of the lower diastasis can improve the midline gap up to 5 cm. This is a minimally invasive alternative to an abdominoplasty in suitable patients.

Care must be taken to not overtreat here in the abdominal region, as a seroma can develop. Overtreatment can also cause fibrosis which can compromise the gliding of the skin surface.

The use of fat grafting in facial, neck, and body contouring is well established [14]. Coleman is considered the father of fat grafting, popularizing the technique in the early 1990s [15]. He notes that the range of "take" of the fat grafts can range from 10 to 90% [16], depending on the technique and postoperative compliance of the recipient. The enhancement of graft take can be achieved by avoiding large-volume injections, by stratifying the fat injections at multiple levels, and by pulsing

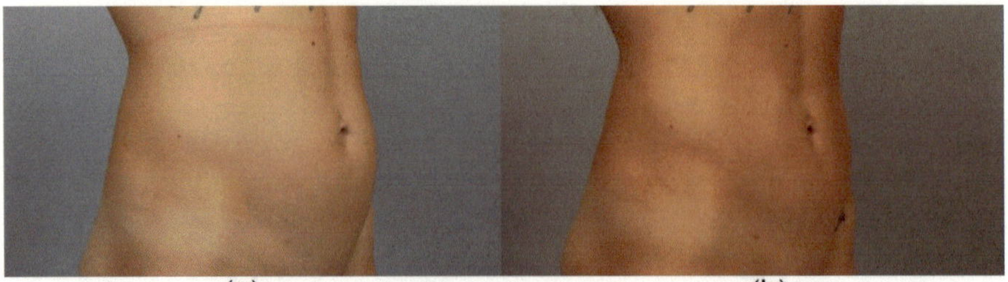

(a) (b)

Figure 8.
(a) 35-year-old mom with diastasis recti. She declined abdominoplasty. (b) 3 months post-Renuvion-assisted liposuction. Significant improvement of her rectus diastasis was obtained.

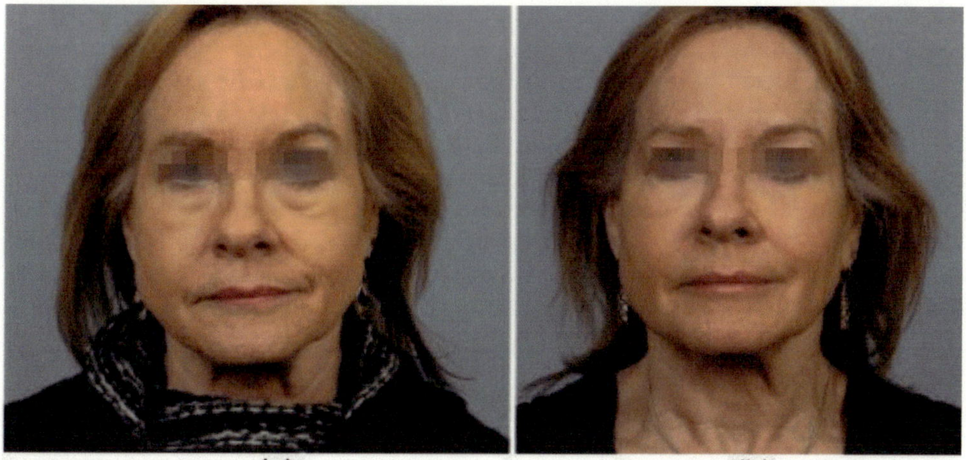

Figure 9.
(a) 58-year-old before treatment. (b) 3 months following laser resurfacing, fat grafting, and intradermal injection of nanofat.

small volumes at a time so that a "string of pearls" effect is achieved. If there is a significant component of liquefied fat in the injectable fat, this will reduce graft take. The traumatized fat or desiccated fat is less viable than the fat harvested at low pressure and kept in a closed container. A current common practice is the topical application of nanofat following nonthermal microneedling, RF microneedling, or fractional laser resurfacing. There is little uptake of progenitor cells with these methods, as the aDSCs are prone to desiccation and traumatic death. A recent publication [17] advocates the use of a biocreme to enhance cell viability. Future development of the novel use of nanofat for skin enhancement will no doubt optimize the technique so that consistent outcomes can be achieved.

An interesting use of nanofat is the injection of the substance intradermally. **Figure 9** shows a patient treated in the infraorbital region using this method. Since the particulate size is very small, the solution can be injected with a 30-gauge needle. The effect of intradermal nanofat improves with time, so that outcomes at 1-year post-injection are much more remarkable than early changes [18]. Regions that can be significantly improved with intradermal nanofat include the upper lip and the infraorbital region. By adding nanofat to the traditional macrofat grafts, the outcomes, especially in facial regions, are enhanced. By milling macrofat into millifat, lumpiness in regions with skin can be reduced.

6. Conclusion

Regenerative medicine has become a popular antiaging resource that patients are actively seeking. Helium plasma-driven fractional radiofrequency energy can restore the lost fibroseptal scaffold in many regions of the face, neck, and body. While FSN contraction can reconstruct a framework of cohesive fatty stroma upon which the skin can rest, aged skin will not be appreciably improved as it is not directly addressed. Instead of using damaging resurfacing techniques such as laser ablation or thermal microneedling, the regenerative restoration of dermal fibroblasts as well as the generation of a new blood supply helps to thicken the dermis as well as improve the tone, texture, and wrinkles. Little downtime is seen with the use of nanofat injections, and there is very little temporary deformity. The addition of nanofat to traditional fat for grafting enhances both structural and vascular response. As with most esthetic procedures, combination therapy is superior to the use of a single modality when an optimal outcome is desired. The use of helium plasma-driven radiofrequency energy for soft tissue contouring and skin tightening is an excellent approach for the restoration of the supportive fibroseptal network. Nanofat plus more traditional approaches can optimize the correction of volume deficiencies as well as the correction of thin, structurally deficient skin. As research and development of both of these techniques evolves, biological restoration of the aging soft tissues is predicted to become more popular than other surgical or injectable approaches.

Author details

Diane Irvine Duncan
Private Practice in Fort Collins, Colorado, USA

*Address all correspondence to: momsurg@aol.com

References

[1] Paul M, Mulholland RS. A new approach for adipose tissue treatment and body contouring using radiofrequency-assisted liposuction. Aesthetic Plastic Surgery. 2009;**33**:687-694

[2] Chen SS, Wright NT, Humphrey JD. Heat-induced changes in the mechanics of a collagenous tissue: Isothermal free shrinkage. Journal of Biomechanical Engineering. 1997;**109**:372-378

[3] Cohen SR, Tiryaki T, et al. Cellular optimization of nanofat: Comparison of two nanofat processing devices in terms of cell count and viability. Aesthetic Surgery Journal Open Forum. December 2019;**1**(4):ojz028. DOI: 10.1093/asjof/ojz028

[4] Duncan DI. Improving outcomes in upper arm liposuction: Adding radiofrequency-assisted liposuction to induce skin contraction. Aesthetic Surgery Journal. 2012;**32**(1):84-95

[5] DiBernardo BE, Reyes J. Evaluation of skin tightening after laser-assisted liposuction. Aesthetic Surgery Journal. 2009;**29**:400-407

[6] McBean J, Katz B. Laser Lipolysis: an update. The Journal of Clinical and Aesthetic Dermatology. 2011;**4**(7):25-34

[7] Tiryaki T. Micro-shuttle lifting of the neck: A percutaneous loop suspension method using a novel double-ended needle. Aesthetic Surgery Journal. 2016;**36**(6):629-638. DOI: 101093/asj/swj001. Epub: 23 February 2016

[8] Hurwitz D et al. Enhancing masculine features after massive weight loss. Aesthetic Plastic Surgery. 2016;**40**:245-255. DOI: 10.1007/s00266-016-0617-x. Published online: 18 February 2016. PMCID: PMC481945

[9] Duncan DI, Dinev I. Noninvasive induction of muscle fiber hypertrophy and hyperplasia: Effects of high-intensity focused electromagnetic field evaluated in an in-vivo porcine model: A pilot study. Aesthetic Surgery Journal. 26 October 2019:sjz244. DOI: 10.1093/asj/sjz244

[10] Cotofana S, Fratila AA, Schenck TL, Redka-Swoboda W, Zilinsky I, Pavicic T. The anatomy of the aging face: A review. Facial Plastic Surgery. 2016;**32**(3):253-260. DOI: 10.1055/s-0036-1582234. Epub: 01 June 2016. Review

[11] Duncan DI. Restoring a pleasant facial expression with minimally invasive techniques. Aesthetic Surgery Journal. 2004;**24**:574-579

[12] Dobke M, Hauch A. Targeting facial aging with nano and regenerative technologies and procedures. Plastic and Aesthetic Research. 2020;**7**:1. DOI: 10.20517/2347-9264.2019.65. Received: 30 November 2019; First Decision: 02 January 2020; Revised: 02 January 2020. https://parjournal.net/article/view/3320

[13] https://www.plasticsurgery.org/documents/News/Statistics/2018/plastic-surgery-statistics-full-report-2018.pdf [Accessed: 21 December 2019]

[14] Kaufman MR, Miller TA, Huang C, et al. Autologous fat transfer for facial recontouring: Is there science behind the art? Plastic and Reconstructive Surgery. 2007;**119**:2287-2296

[15] Coleman SR et al. Facial recontouring with lipostructure. Clinics in Plastic Surgery. 1997;**24**:347-367

[16] Strong AL, Cederna PS, et al. The current state of fat grafting: A review of harvesting, processing, and injection

techniques. Plastic and Reconstructive Surgery. 2015;**136**(4):912. DOI: 10.1097/PRS.0000000000001590. PMCID: PMC4833505. Author manuscript; available in PMC October 1, 2016; Published in final edited form as: Plast Reconstr Surg. 2015; 897-913

[17] Cohen SR. Topical nanofat biocrème improves aesthetic outcomes of nonablative fractionated laser treatment: A preliminary report. Aesthetic Surgery Journal. 05 September 2019:sjz240. DOI: 10.1093/asj/sjz240

[18] Trivisonno A, Alexander R, et al. Intraoperative Strategies for minimal manipulation of autologous adipose tissue for cell- and tissue-based therapies: Concise review. Stem Cells Translational Medicine. 2019;**8**(12):1265-1271. DOI: 10.1002/sctm.19-0166. PMCID: PMC6877766

Chapter 5

Combining PDO Threads with Exosomes for Microlifting

Diane Irvine Duncan

Abstract

A recent survey of practicing plastic surgeons showed that regenerative medicine is the current top interest of esthetic consumers worldwide. Patients are frequently requesting correction of small regions, instead of opting for an all-encompassing procedure associated with prolonged recovery time. Thus, the field of "microlifting" has emerged. This is a new approach in which minimally invasive procedures can be utilized to accomplish outcomes formerly reserved for traditional surgery. The combination of polydioxanone (PDO) threads and topical exosomes is a method of treating both underlying soft tissue laxity and the surface of aging skin. The application of exosomes can deliver topical growth factors and targeted peptides to assist in rapid skin surface healing. More than a simple delivery vesicle, exosomes communicate with cells at the recipient site and can induce cellular change. PDO threads can be used subcutaneously as both a suspension device and regenerative biostimulatory device. Usually resorbed at 6 months post-insertion, these threads leave behind a linear network of collagen and elastin fibers that remains long after the polydioxanone is gone. Combination therapies can target several concerns when performed simultaneously. This regenerative method is well accepted by patients due to minimal cost and recovery time.

Keywords: injectable implant, threadlift, exosomes, particulate drug delivery, growth factors, PDO threads, filler threads

1. Introduction

The number of practitioners joining the esthetic field is increasing rapidly. These specialists range in background and training from aestheticians, chiropractors, and acupuncturists to dentists, dermatologists, facial plastic, and plastic surgeons. While more patients are seeking treatment for concerns regarding facial and body region challenges, few desire traditional surgical intervention with the associated risk and recovery time. Regional differences dictate the preferences of the clientele, but many do seek the restoration of their own youthful appearance instead of a drastic change. In years past, the emergence of stem cell therapy has been viewed by many as a magic wand that could restore aging tissues to a youthful state without surgical intervention. Some limitations to treatment with mesenchymal stem cells (MSCs) include a low survival rate, tumorigenicity, poor "take," and lack of efficacy [1]. It is thought that many of the supposed effects of mesenchymal stem cells are indeed paracrine effects, mediated by acellular factors that are transmitted with the cells, but not by direct effects of the cells themselves [2]. For several years, filler companies have focused on biostimulatory effects seen after the hyaluronic acid, hydroxyapatite, or other fillers have been metabolized [3, 4]. The injectable poly-L-lactic acid works on this principle. A problem can occur when so much filler has been injected that the response turns from collagen stimulation to fibrosis. Some long-term injectable patients note a "woody" or stiff feeling, difficulty achieving a natural animated expression, and chronic swelling in a treatment region years after the original product was injected. A preferred solution would be induction of an existing tissue response using regenerative options now available and in development. Restoration of dermal thickness, collagen, and elastin and self-repair of the adipose framework upon which the skin rests are concepts that make sense to our esthetic customer base.

2. Background

Exosomes, also known as secretomes [5], are formed within the cell from multivesicular endosomes. Intracellular endosomes contain multiple small vesicles measuring 20–200 nm. These multivesicular bodies fuse with the cellular plasma membrane, and exocytosis releases spherical particulate carriers now identified as exosomes. These acellular bilamellar structures contain miRNA, mRNA, and peptides. Exosomes are identified by biomarkers CD9, CD63, CD81, Alix, Tsg101, and flotillin-1. The production of exosomes in a laboratory involves the use of conditioned media (CM) in a cell culture setting. Usually MSCs are the cells cultured. Exosomes can express characteristics of the cells of origin, so directed wound care exosomes might be harvested from conditioned media used in a co-culture of dermal fibroblasts and adipose-derived stem cells (ADSCs). Cell-to-cell communication currently appears to be more important in achieving a desired effect than in achieving the direct effect of MSCs themselves [6]. An example of this has been seen in a co-culture of dermal fibroblasts and mesenchymal stem cells. The formation of "nanotunnels" from cell to cell is seen, so cell signaling is somewhat direct. The ability to transfer information can also be seen with the endosome/exosome route [7]. Transfection of gene products or small peptides through the lipid bilayer of the exosome to recipient cells can induce those cells to change cellular characteristics [8]. STAT3 is found in exosomes and promotes angiogenesis, improves fibroblast proliferation, and decreases the amount of time needed to heal an injury [9]. In regenerative medicine, it has been noted that paracrine signaling can generate up to 91% of the effects of injected stem cells [10]. Thus, the use of exosomes obtained from conditioned media used in cell culture has rapidly become popular in many specialties including cardiology, orthopedics, oncology, and the esthetic field [11]. Esthetic applications include topical application following nonthermal microneedling, RF microneedling, fractional laser resurfacing, and plasma-driven resurfacing. In these instances, reduction of downtime and improvement in skin tone and texture have been noted [12]. The FDA issued a statement [13] in December 2019 that, as yet, no exosomes have been cleared by the agency; therefore, topical use only is advised. Because the product is acellular, many companies producing these products note that they are exempt from FDA scrutiny or GMP manufacturing processes. However, since the FDA classifies any biological that is intended to penetrate the stratum corneum in order to change the structure or function of any aspect of the human body as a drug, practitioners who inject exosomes are violating FDA guidelines [14].

Polydioxanone (PDO) threads have become popular worldwide over a period of approximately 5 years. These threads can be used in place of fillers for such purposes as dorsal nasal augmentation, improvement of deep dermal or superficial hypodermal defects, and focal depressions. Improvement of skin laxity by using barbed threads as suspension devices is also growing again in popularity. While barbed threads originated more than 20 years ago, the early devices were created by hand cutting existing sutures, creating a weak spot at the base of the cut in the thinnest area of the suture diameter. Early threads were notorious for breakage, extrusion, and "cheese wiring" or cutting through soft tissue to extrude through the skin [15]. The "lunchtime facelift" was performed using percutaneous threads that could create bunching and superficial contour irregularities. Patients noted either little result in many cases or complained about the lack of longevity. The use of permanent sutures resulted in a mixture of good and not so good results. This history parallels that of permanent fillers: an irreversible outcome has no easy solution if a problem arises [16]. Thus, many practitioners are now choosing threads that are resorbable over time.

Because regeneration of the subcutaneous layer is as important as skin rejuvenation, the emphasis on biostimulatory products has increased during recent years. Erosion of the collagen matrix that binds the adipose framework supporting the overlying skin has been well documented (**Figure 1**). Restoration of the collagen and elastin fraction of the fibroseptal network has been noted primarily with radiofrequency-assisted soft tissue stimulation [17]. Poly-L-lactic acid can also stimulate collagen formation over time. Because it is sometimes difficult to get the compound into solution and because it is somewhat expensive to the consumer, widespread adoption of this injectable has lagged behind acceptance of HA and hydroxylapatite fillers. Late granuloma formation is also a deterrent to its use [18]. First popularized in Asia, PDO (polydioxanone) threads [19] have been rapidly accepted in that part of the world. Advantages include longevity similar to that of fillers with a significantly lower product cost. Ease of administration is a plus, and the lack of intravascular accidents due to the mechanics of threads offers a superior safety profile. PDO threads are available in several styles. "Mono" threads are used in the deep dermis or in the superficial hypodermis. They are usually injected in a stacked pattern (nasal dorsum) for filling volume-deficient regions. They can also be placed in a crosshatched "woven" pattern to stimulate soft tissue neocollagenesis in a pattern similar to that of Sculptra. The effect of small diameter threads can be subtle, but these are excellent for use in patients with very thin skin.

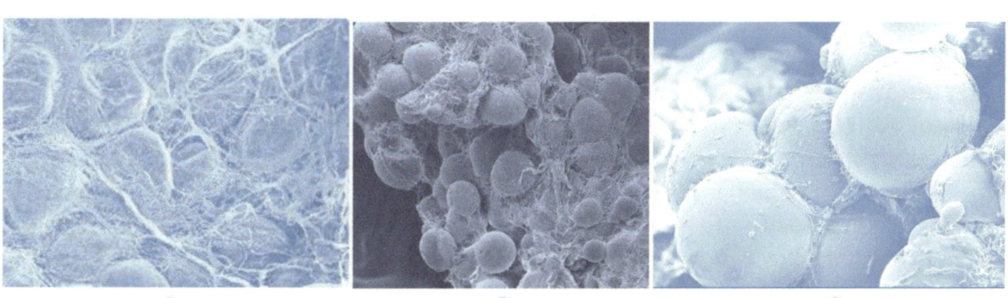

Figure 1.
Scanning electron micrographs of aging adipose tissue. (A) A 23-year-old shows a dense three-dimensional "net" of collagenous stroma forming a scaffold that holds adipose cells in a firm and defined shape. (B) In middle age an irregular erosion of this framework is apparent. (C) A 61-year-old patient shows complete loss of the fibroseptal network that shapes and supports the subcutaneous adipose layer.

Early manufacture of barbed threads involved several cuts after manufacturing of the suture, but this can cause weak points as noted, and therefore breakage can be problematic. Molded threads retain their central integrity, so tensile strength is improved. Cogs or cones can be used instead of or in addition to barbs in order to secure tissue attachment. A new double-coated polydioxanone thread combines these two modalities in order to strongly secure soft tissue. These threads have a 2-year effect; when the outer layer erodes and resorbs, the inner thread remains intact.

A new thread type unique to the Miracu (Mission Viejo, CA) company is known as Meshfill TM. These filler threads consist of 16 tiny woven PDO threads formed into a hollow cylinder. They can be used alone or in combination with fat or filler. When filled with the correct amount of complementary filler, the product can be contained in the cylinder's space. Meshfill can be stacked in area needing more volume, such as the cheeks or chin. When used with autologous fat transfer, the volume correction is retained as the fat becomes newly vascularized. Meshfill can be used in difficult-to-treat regions such as the infraorbital region and oral commissures.

3. Materials and methods

Topical exosomes are available in the USA from several commercial producers. Benev (Mission Viejo, CA) currently offers the most cost-effective version. Because the FDA considers any formulation intended to change the structure or function of a human that is administered deeper than the stratum corneum [14], the use of exosomes is now limited to cosmetic use as a topical application. The Benev formulation consists of two vials. One vial contains lyophilized exosomes that are to be reconstituted and are obtained from progenitor cells treated with conditioned media. The second vial of diluent contains hyaluronic acid, which is a strong hydrator, plus multiple growth factors and small peptides. Once mixed, the preparation should be refrigerated. The solution can be applied topically to the skin on label. Exosomes are also used following treatment with microneedling, nitrogen plasma resurfacing, application of radiofrequency energy, fractional laser, and dermaplaning in order to optimize rapid healing. Ideally several serial applications should be made in order to obtain the most benefit.

PDO threads can be added to the skin treatment in order to improve the tone and laxity of the subcutaneous layer. The biostimulatory nature of PDO threads is seen in **Figure 2**. A small collagenous tunnel develops over 1 month, surrounding the thread as it gradually resorbs. This soft tissue support remains after the thread itself disappears. Most esthetic practitioners employ combination treatments in order to optimize outcomes for their aging patients, as a single solution generally does not address all defects. Three areas of subcutaneous improvement can be targeted. Problems addressed include mild to moderate soft tissue atrophy; this type of defect may be best treated with mono threads. Soft tissue laxity and mild to moderate pendulosity of the jowls and nasolabial folds are usually addressed with barbed threads. The longer lasting threads are recommended for use by skilled practitioners as these can be difficult to remove. Focal volumetric defects such as prejowl sulcus, gonial notching, a retrusive chin, drooping oral commissures, infraorbital hollowing, and the depression associated with malar bags all respond well to Meshfill injection. Excellent correction of deep nasolabial folds is also seen with Meshfill.

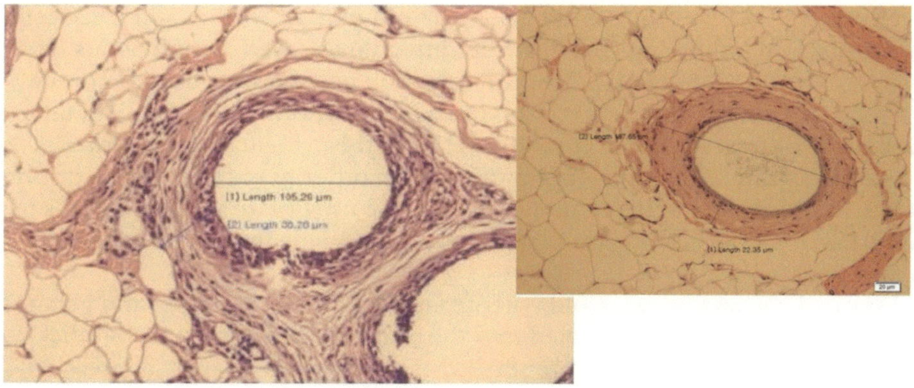

Figure 2.
Polydioxanone thread hollow and granulation tissue with newly made collagen fibers, 1 month after thread insertion, White Yucatan pig study. Source: Research by Yonsei Clinical Medicine Research Center, Dr. Junghyun Yoon, and Dr. Sangseob Kim with N-Finders Co., Ltd.

The patient should be marked in the upright position prior to thread insertion. Injection can be performed either upright or in a semirecumbent position. However, when tightening barbed threads, this is best done while the patient is upright. Markings are performed with a brow pencil prior to thread insertion. The vector of tightening is calculated. Generally, two or three threads are needed per region for optimal effect. Application of topical anesthesia prior to treatment is routinely performed. Removal of the topical anesthetic along with sterile prep and drape is the standard of care. Hair is contained so that thread contact is minimized. While mono threads are commonly injected without local anesthetic, a small amount of intradermal local anesthesia greatly improves patient comfort. With barbed thread insertion and Meshfill injection, it is recommended to numb both the insertion site and the line or track along which the thread will be placed. Only a small amount of lidocaine is needed per region. The use of 0.5 or 1% lidocaine with epinephrine will minimize bruising if injected in full 3 minutes prior to thread insertion. An insertion point for the cannula is placed approximately 0.5–1 cm proximal to the region to be filled. Thus, the thread should be held in place over the treatment target prior to choosing an access point, in order to be sure the thread length is correct. The importance of this point cannot be overstated. If not injected well beyond the actual treatment target, threads can migrate, and the ends can create a superficial deformity.

4. Results

Combination therapy, especially when performing microlifting, generally produces a more profound improvement than when using a single treatment modality. Triple treatments for face and neck rejuvenation in patients seeking minimal recovery time include light fractional resurfacing or nitrogen plasma resurfacing, application of exosomes to the treatment region for enhanced outcome and rapid healing, and volumization and tissue suspension with PDO threads. In many states, these treatments can be delegated to a licensed supervised provider.

It is recommended that only skilled physicians inject Meshfill or Line threads, as the treating provider should be able to take care of any potential complication that might occur.

Figure 3 illustrates the case of a 56-year-old patient who sought treatment for infraorbital hollowing. She had filler injections as well as autologous fat grafting. Her result following Meshfill injection plus fat introduced into the cylinder shows a dramatic correction in an area that is historically difficult to treat. Meshfill insertion in this region is below the orbicularis muscle at the level of the orbital rim. A 30 mm length was used in order to reduce the risk of thread visibility. In patients with lateral hollowing, the use of two shorter threads per region can yield more accurate placement than a single longer thread in this curved region.

Figure 4 shows a 74-year-old with drooping oral commissures and general volume loss. Meshfill was injected into the oral commissures in an "X" distribution so that the threads were stacked at the point of deepest depression. 30 mm threads were used at this location in combination with 0.2 cc Restylane

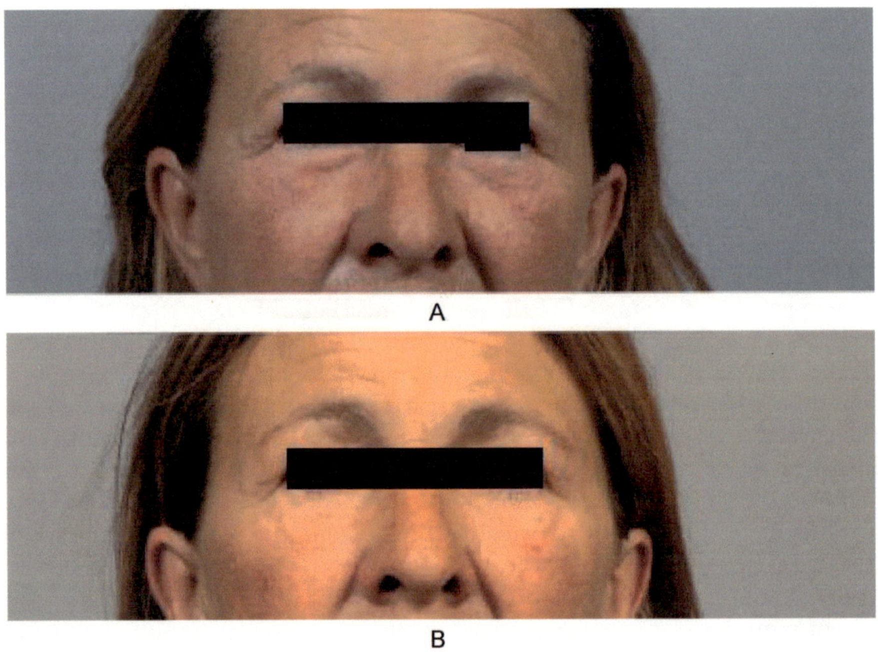

Figure 3.
(A) A 56-year-old patient before treatment. Previous infraorbital treatments included filler and fat grafting. (B) The same patient 2 weeks postinjection of Meshfill PDO cylinders plus 0.2 cc hyaluronic acid filler per side.

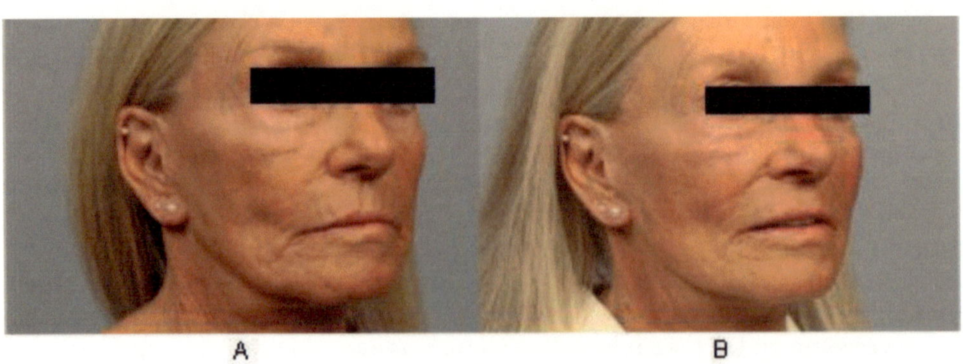

Figure 4.
(A) A 74-year-old patient with age-related soft tissue atrophy. (B) Two-week postinjection of Meshfill plus intraluminal injection of 0.2–0.3 cc HA filler per site: Cheeks, perioral, and infraorbital regions.

per injection site. 40 mm Meshfill was stacked in the malar region in order to achieve volumetric enhancement.

Figure 5 denotes a 53-year-old patient treated with a combination of barbed threads and Meshfill in the brow region. The often flat supraorbital rim can be contoured and lifted using this unique combination (**Figure 6**).

Figure 7 depicts the improvement in rapidity of healing that can be achieved by applying topical exosomes. Normally, fully ablative erbium laser resurfacing takes 7–10 days to fully re-epithelialize. This patient had full skin surface repopulation in 5 days. Application of exosomes, then Aquaphor ointment, was performed twice a day for 2 days.

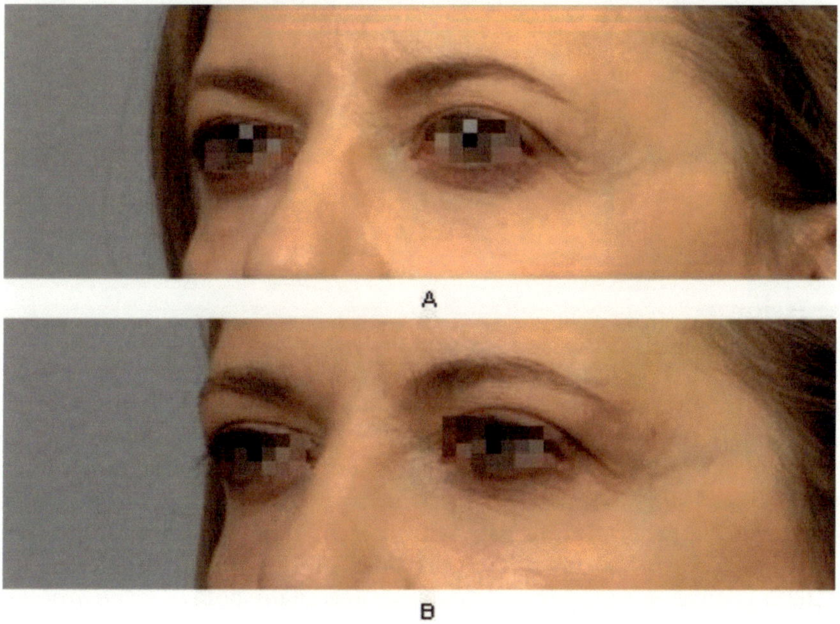

Figure 5.
(A) A 53-year-old patient noting a flattening of the supraorbital rim and loss of brow structure. (B) Two-week post-insertion of two PDO barbed threads per lateral brow plus injection of Meshfill and 0.3 cc HA filler underneath the brow itself.

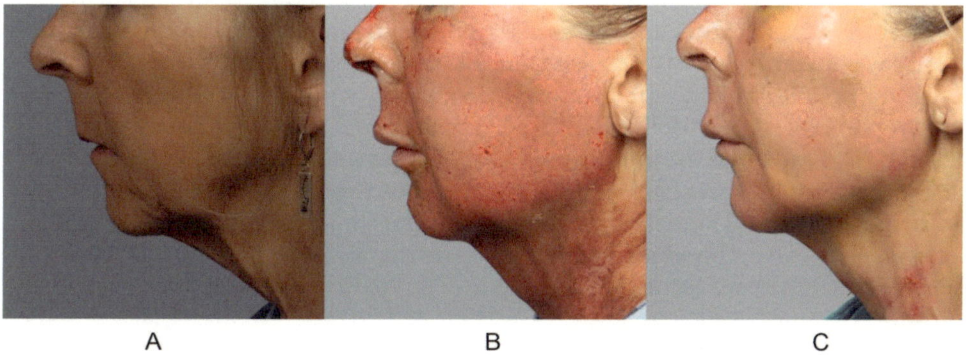

Figure 6.
(A) A 75-year-old before RF needling, laser resurfacing, fat grafting, and exosome application. (B) Two days post-treatment, most areas have re-epithelialized. Usually this process takes 6–8 days. (C) One month post-treatment, the patient's facial contour and jawline has changed dramatically. No surgical facelift was performed.

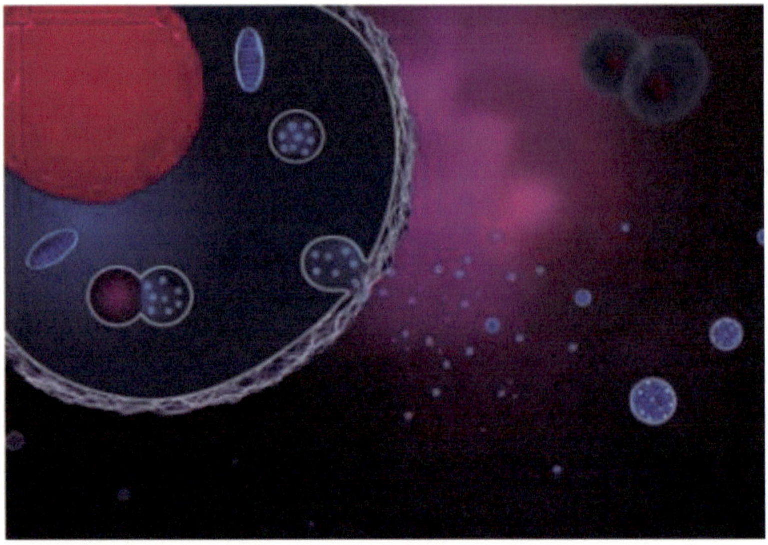

Figure 7.
Diagram of intracellular exosomes.

5. Discussion

Botulinum toxin and fillers have been the standard introductory maintenance treatment for the improvement of age-related lines and volumetric lines for many years. "Filler fatigue" is a growing phenomenon, especially when the cost of treatment is calculated. As with any repeated procedure, the cost is not only monetary. For most patients, time spent recovering from a procedure, which limits their ability to work or enjoy leisure activities, is a real concern. Many tend to choose a lesser procedure based solely on "down" time. The lack of longevity with filler and toxin injections is a common complaint. As patients age, many note that the problem they are experiencing cannot be adequately addressed with these two types of injections. Regenerative options are being sought as an alternative to standard approaches, as restoration of one's own tissues is preferred to injecting toxins or foreign substances. Microlifting [20], a term coined by Tiryaki, is an approach that generally combines subcutaneous thread placement with other regenerative approaches.

While stem cell therapy is regarded as the highest form of regenerative medicine, recent research disputes that conventional wisdom. Many papers in different specialties note that cell-to-cell signaling has much more of an effect at the treatment target than the progenitor cells themselves do [21]. Exosomes are present in all tissues. They are formed when endosomes, or intracellular multivesicular particles, fuse with the cell's plasma membrane. Smaller nanoparticulate vesicles "bud out" into the intercellular space (**Figure 8**). Exosomes are able to communicate with other cells without making direct contact. In the early 1980s, exosomes were thought to be a receptacle for intracellular waste. Named in 1987, exosomes [22] were found to be the messengers that transfer behavior instructions to a recipient cell located in the region. The "paracrine effect" is the way that exosomes communicate with target cells (**Figure 7**). These nanoparticles generally measure 20–100 microns and less than 0.1 micron. They reside within endosomes, which are multivesicular organelles located within the cell. After binding with the internal plasma membrane, these nanoparticles are released outside the cell. Able to communicate with multiple cells in the region, exosomes are capable of inducing a change in behavior of a nearby cell without depending on direct cell contact.

They contain messenger RNA, microRNA, proteins, lipids, cytokines, bioactive compounds, and nucleic acids [23]. **Figure 9** shows the formation of exosomes from intracellular endosomes. Exosomes have been shown to promote proliferation of the target cell and more rapid healing than with a PBS buffer or depleted media in vitro [24]. Repair of injury with exosomes was noted to be three times as fast as the injury

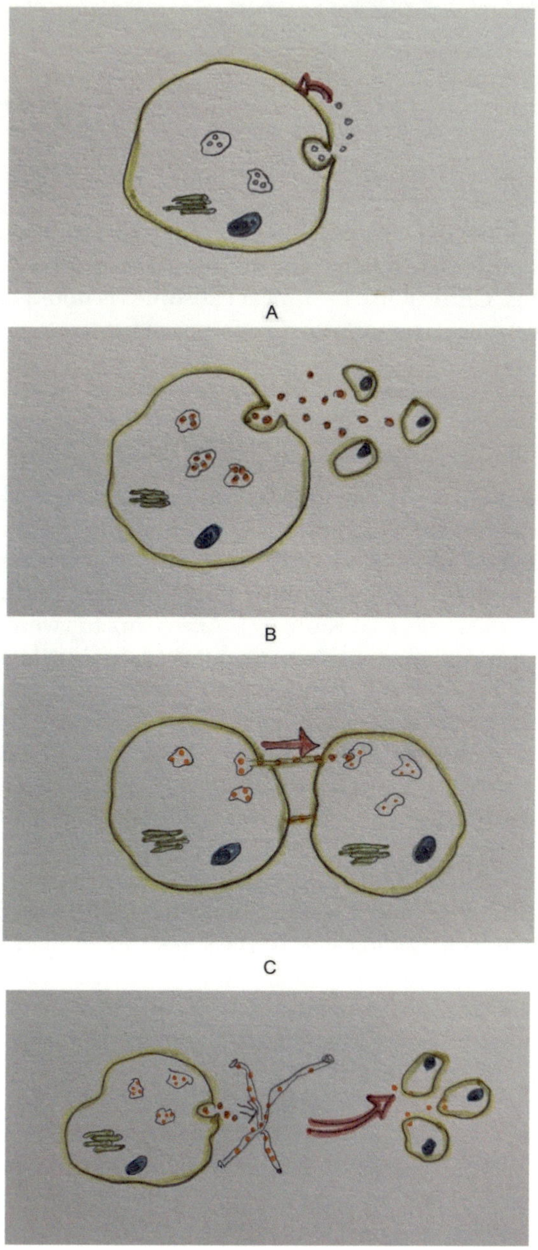

Figure 8.
(A) Autrocrine signaling occurs when intracellularly derived particles influence the same cell at the extracellular membrane level. (B) Paracrine signaling occurs when exosomes are released into the extracellular fluid, thus influencing the behavior of cells within the local region. (C) Direct cell to cell communication can occur when adjacent cells build nanotunnels through which intracellular proteins and RNA is shared. (D) Endocrine signaling occurs when a substance such as a hormone enters the nearby bloodstream, influencing cellular behavior in a distant location.

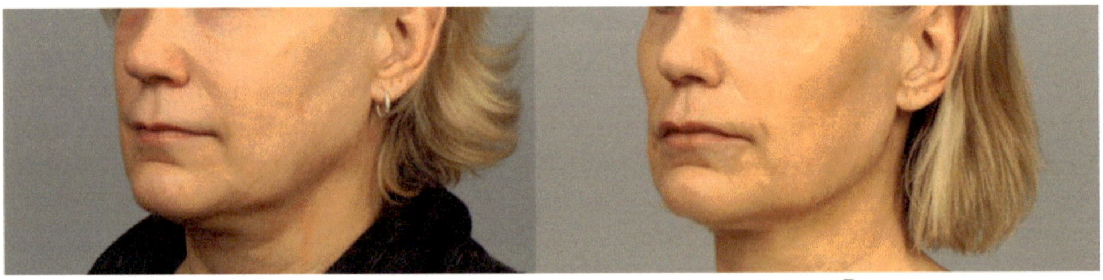

Figure 9.
Clinical effect of exosomes. (A) A 62-year-old patient 2 days following ablative erbium laser resurfacing. (B) The same patient on day 5. Usually these patients require 7–10 days of healing in order to achieve re-epithelialization.

treated with buffer alone and two times as fast as the region treated with depleted media. The response was dose related; the dose of 10 mcg/ml seemed optimal in laboratory conditions. Clinical use of topical exosomes is noted to improve healing in patients who undergo fractional resurfacing procedures.

6. PDO threads

Alcamo was the first to use barbed threads and is given credit for his invention in 1964 [25]. These threads were hand cut and barbs were unidirectional. MacKenzie [26] is credited with the development of the bidirectional barbed thread. In the late 1980s, Sulamanidze noted the use of modified polypropylene sutures for subcutaneous facial lifting without skin excision [27]. Aptos threads were developed and became popular for improving soft tissue pendulosity since little downtime was required. While some patients experienced good results, many major complications were reported, including breakage, rippling, facial distortion, extrusion, infection, and cheese wiring of the suture through the skin [28]. Wu [29] developed his own version of a barbed thread and noted that all effects were lost over time; patients needed to repeat the procedure in order to retain benefit. Ruff was awarded a patent for developing a barbed thread in 1994, with his first prototype a weed whacker cord [30]. FDA clearance in the USA was achieved in 2004, when a polypropylene, then later a polydioxanone device, was developed by Quill. Shortly thereafter, the contour thread was withdrawn from the market. At the time, threads had attained some notoriety due to a combination of use by poorly trained individuals and a rash of publicized complications. Threads have made a bit of a comeback, as better training and safer resorbable sutures are being introduced. Currently there are several remaining barbed sutures available in US origin. Stratafix, a permanent barbed suture by Ethicon, has been discontinued in practice due to the intense fibrotic response and patient complaints of inflammation and discomfort in the treatment region. V-lock is resorbable and seems better tolerated, especially in breast surgery. Silhouette is FDA cleared for midface lifting [30] and also claims to be biostimulatory [31]. Since 2015, several companies have applied for FDA clearance of their polydioxanone threads for the approximation of the skin. Miracu threads [32] have received FDA clearance for both the PDO thread and the cannula insertion device.

Many styles of PDO threads are available. Filler threads have no fixation and are intended to supply a small amount of volume as well as hypodermal stimulation. Bidirectional barbed threads can be placed with a needle from the center of the treatment region. An alternative is the placement of these threads from within a cannula which avoids a central puncture mark. “Spring” threads are used in areas where dynamic motion is prominent and might be restricted with a linear model. The novel Meshfill device (**Figure 10**) is a cylinder made of 16 tiny woven PDO threads that is inserted within a cannula. Prior to cannula withdrawal, 0.2 cc of either filler or fat can be injected into the internal space. The concept of an injectable implant has a great utility. In regions where a firm or defined contour is needed—the chin, cheek, or jawline, for example—these devices can be stacked or lined up to dramatically enhance shape. In regions where a linear depression is noted—the nasolabial fold—dramatic rather than subtle correction can be obtained with a very small amount of additional filler or fat.

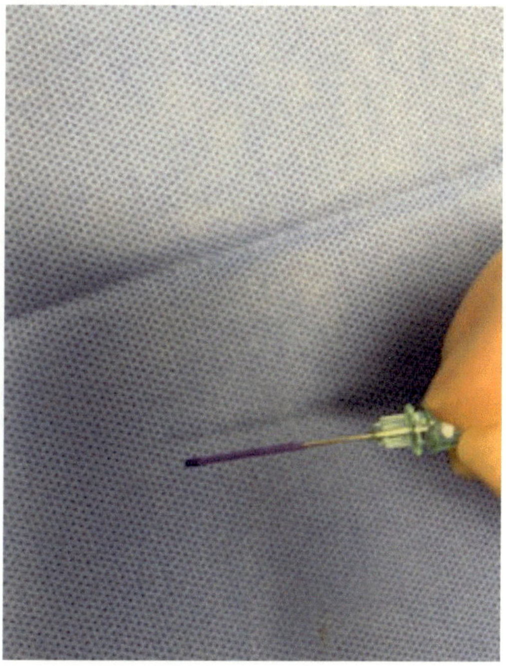

Figure 10.
Diagram of Meshfill construction. Sixteen tiny PDO threads are woven and placed on a 21 gauge cannula. These cylindrical structures can be used as filler threads by themselves or can be filled with fat or fillers to augment the volumetric correction.

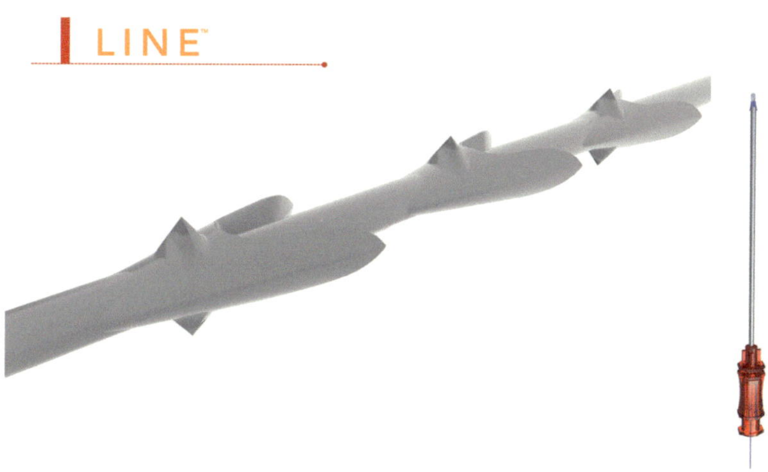

Figure 11.
Miracu line thread. This PDO thread employs barbs and cogs in a double-coated structure that lasts up to 2 years.

A new addition to the portfolio is a double-coated PDO thread that combined barbs and cogs. The Miracu Line TM device is molded, not cut, so there is no weak point along the thread (**Figure 11**). The thread called "Line" lasts for 2 years. As the outer coating is resorbed, the inner thread maintains a presence and continues to offer soft tissue support. Because of the semipermanent nature of the Line thread, it is recommended that only skilled physicians use the device, with care taken to place it deep enough so that a contour defect is avoided. Manipulation of these threads should not be overdone as they are difficult to remove.

7. Conclusion

While patient acceptance of injectables has been high, many educated consumers are now seeking regenerative solutions for their esthetic needs. Combination treatment of the skin and subcutaneous stromal scaffold is attractive to both patients and physicians. The use of exosomes to signal cells in the treatment region is a rapidly growing trend. When combined with a light resurfacing protocol, exosomes accelerate the healing process while delivering mRNA, cytokines, chemokines, and growth factors. Restoration of the support system of the skin, the subcutaneous stroma, can be enhanced with PDO resorbable threads that are biostimulatory. Mono threads will generate directional collagen ingrowth in the superficial hypodermis. Barbed suspension threads can support sagging regions. Cylinder configured threads can be used alone or in combination with filler or fat. These injectable implants can replace small surgically introduced facial implants in many cases. Microlifting using suspension threads combined with regenerative techniques is a popular alternative to traditional injectable techniques.

Author details

Diane Irvine Duncan
Private Practice, Fort Collins, Colorado, USA

*Address all correspondence to: momsurg@aol.com

References

[1] Knoepfler PS. Deconstructing stem cell tumorigenicity: A roadmap to safe regenerative medicine. Stem Cells. 2009;**27**(5):1050-1056. DOI: 10.1002/stem.37. PMCID: PMC2733374

[2] Gurunathan S et al. Review of the isolation, characterization, biological function, and multifarious therapeutic approaches of exosomes. Cell. 2019;**8**(4):307. DOI: 10.3390/cells8040307. PMCID: PMC6523673

[3] De Almeida AT, Figuerdo V, et al. Consensus recommendations for the use of hyperdiluted calcium hydroxyapatite (Radiesse) as a face and body biostimulatory agent. Plastic and Reconstructive Surgery. Global Open. 2019;**7**(3):e2160. DOI: 10.1097/GOX.0000000000002160. PMCID: PMC6467620

[4] Amselem M. Radiesse®: A novel rejuvenation treatment for the upper arms. Clinical, Cosmetic and Investigational Dermatology. 2016;**9**:9-14. DOI: 10.2147/CCID.S93137. PMCID: PMC4699473

[5] Mitchell R, Mellows B, Sheard J, et al. Secretome of adipose-derived mesenchymal stem cells promotes skeletal muscle regeneration through synergistic action of extracellular vesicle cargo and soluble proteins. Stem Cell Research & Therapy. 2019;**10**:116. DOI: 10.1186/s13287-019-1213-1. PMCID: PMC6451311

[6] Ferraris V. How do cells talk to each other? Paracrine factors secreted by mesenchymal stromal cells. The Journal of Thoracic and Cardiovascular Surgery. 2016;**151**(3):849-851. DOI: 10.1016/j.jtcvs.2015.11.035. [Epub: 27 November 2015]

[7] Rustom A, Saffrich R, Markovic I, Walther P, Gerdes HH. Nanotubular highways for intercellular organelle transport. Science. 2004;**303**:1007-1010

[8] Poe AJ, Knowlton AA. Exosomes as agents of change in the cardiovascular system. Journal of Molecular and Cellular Cardiology. 2017;**111**:40-50. DOI: 10.1016/j.yjmcc.2017.08.002

[9] Shabbir A, Cox A, et al. Mesenchymal cell exosomes include proliferation and migration of normal and chronic wound fibroblasts, and enhance angiogenesis in vitro. Stem Cells and Development. 2015;**24**(14):1635-1647. DOI: 10.1089/scd. 2014.0316. [Epub: 13 April 2015]

[10] van Balkom BW, de Jong OG, Smits M, Brummelman J, den Ouden K, de Bree PM, et al. Endothelial cells require miR-214 to secrete exosomes that suppress senescence and induce angiogenesis in human and mouse endothelial cells. Blood. 2013;**121**:3997-4006; S1-S15

[11] Rashed MH, Bayraktar E, Helal G, et al. Exosomes: From garbage bins to promising therapeutic targets. International Journal of Molecular Sciences. 2017;**18**(3):538. DOI: 10.3390/ijms18030538. PMCID: PMC5372554

[12] Hu L, Wang J, Zhou X, et al. Exosomes derived from human adipose mesenchymal stem cells accelerates cutaneous wound healing via optimizing the characteristics of fibroblasts. Scientific Reports. 2016;**6**:32993. DOI: 10.1038/srep32993. PMCID: PMC5018733

[13] https://www.fda.gov/vaccines-blood-biologics/safety-availability-biologics/public-safety-notification-exosome-products [Accessed: 20 December 2019]

[14] https://www.fda.gov/regulatory-information/search-fda-guidance-documents/regulatory-considerations-microneedling-devices [Accessed: 21 September 2018]

[15] Rakesh K. Use of barbed threads in facial rejuvenation. Indian Journal of Plastic Surgery. 2008;**41**(Suppl):S93-S100

[16] Fukaya M. Long-term effect of the insoluble thread-lifting technique. Clinical, Cosmetic and Investigational Dermatology. 2017;**10**:483-491. DOI: 10.2147/CCID.S150738. PMCID: PMC5697446

[17] Duncan DI. Nonexcisional tissue tightening: Creating skin surface area reduction during abdominal liposuction by adding radiofrequency heating. Aesthetic Surgery Journal. 2013;**8**:1154-1166

[18] Storer M, Euwer R, Calame A, Kourosh S. Late-onset granuloma formation after poly-l-lactic acid injection. JAAD Case Reports. 2016;**2**(1):54-56. DOI: 10.1016/j.jdcr.2015.11.017. PMCID: PMC4809477

[19] Tang S, Sun Z, Wu X, Wang YY, Zhang J. An innovative thread-lift technique for facial rejuvenation and complication management: A Case Report. Medicine (Baltimore). 2018;**97**(21):e10547. DOI: 10.1097/MD.0000000000010547

[20] Tiryaki T. Micro-shuttle lifting of the neck: A percutaneous loop suspension method using a novel double-ended needle. Aesthetic Surgery Journal. 2016;**36**(6):629-638. DOI: 101093/asj/swj001. [Epub: 23 February 2006]

[21] Wang Y, Pennock S, Chen X, Wang Z. Endosomal signaling of epidermal growth factor receptor stimulates signal transduction pathways leading to cell survival. Molecular and Cellular Biology. 2002;**22**(20):7279-7290. DOI: 10.1128/MCB.22.20.7279-7290.2002. PMCID: PMC139821

[22] Johnstone RM, Adam M, Hammond JR, Orr L, Turbide C. Vesicle formation during reticulocyte maturation. Association of plasma membrane activities with released vesicles (exosomes). The Journal of Biological Chemistry. 1987;**262**:9412-9420

[23] Théry C, Amigorena S, Raposo G, Clayton A. Isolation and characterization of exosomes from cell culture supernatants and biological fluids. Current Protocols in Cell Biology. 2006;**3**(3):22

[24] Cui X, He Z, Liang Z, Chen Z, Wang H, Zhang J. Exosomes from adipose-derived mesenchymal stem cells protect the myocardium against ischemia/reperfusion injury through Wnt/β-catenin signaling pathway. Journal of Cardiovascular Pharmacology. 2017;**70**(4):225-231. DOI: 10.1097/FJC.0000000000000507

[25] Alcamo J. US Patent # 3,123,077; 1964. Available from: https://patents.google.com/patent/US3123077A/en [Accessed: 12 October 2019]

[26] MacKenzie A. An experimental multiple barbed suture for the long flexor tendons of the palms and fingers. JBJS British Volume. 1964;**498**(3):440-447

[27] Sulamanidze MA, Fournier PF, Paikidze TG, Sulamanidze GM. Removal of facial soft tissue ptosis with special threads. Dermatologic Surgery. 2002;**28**(5):367-373

[28] Bertossi D, Botti G, Gualdi A, et al. Effectiveness, longevity, and complications of facelift by barbed suture insertion. Aesthetic Surgery Journal. 2019;**39**(3):241-247

[29] Wu WTL. Commentary on: Effectiveness, longevity, and complications of facelift by barbed suture insertion. Aesthetic Surgery Journal. 2019;**39**(3):248-253. DOI: 10.1093/asj/sjy340. PMCID: PMC6376340

[30] Ruff GL. Inserting device foe a barbed tissue connector. US Patent No. 5342376; 1994

[31] https://www.accessdata.fda.gov/scrIpts/cdrh/cfdocs/cfRL/rl.cfm?start_search=1&OwnerOperatorNumber=10032162 [Accessed: 20 December 2019]

[32] Consilglio F, Pizzamiglio R, et al. Suture with resorbable cones: Histology and physico-mechanical features. Aesthetic Surgery Journal. 2016;**36**(3):NP122-NP127. DOI: 10.1093/asj/sjv202. PMCID: PMC5127481